From **There** to **Hear**
A Journey Out of Silence

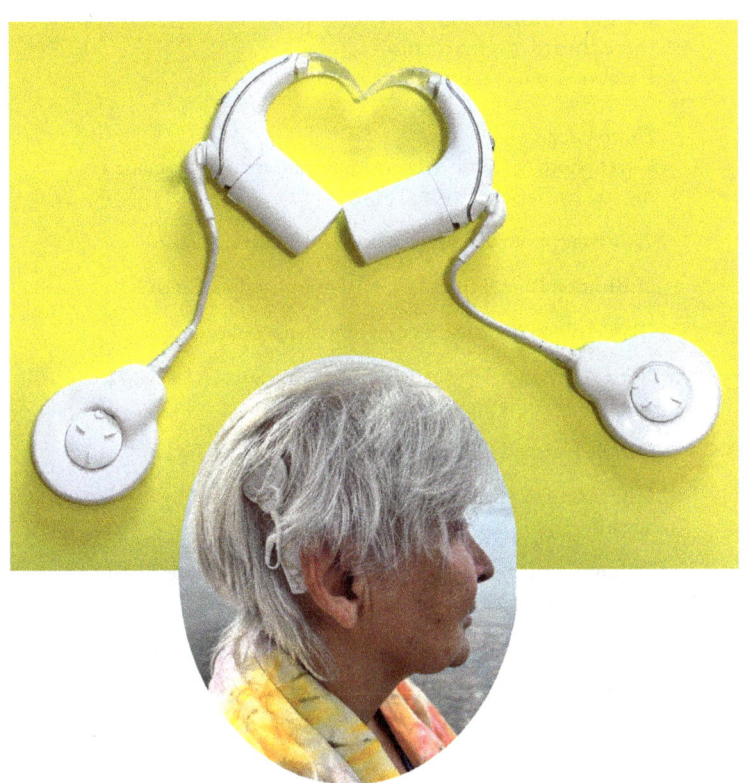

by Carol Rose

Copyright @ 2023 Carol Rose
All rights reserved, including the right of reproduction in whole or in part in any form or technology.
Cover and interior design by Smythtype Design

ISBN: 979-8-218-25723-1

Contact information:
there2hear81@gmail.com
Facebook page From There to Hear

Photo Credits:
Cover photo of Carol "I didn't know butterfly wings made a sound," by Darlene Basto

Title Page photo of Carol's processor by Darlene Basto

Dedication Page, Tenley and Adalyn by Chelsea Green

"Processor on Bandage" Page 34 by Mena Anderson

"First Activation," Page 37, and "Toasting Success," Page 42 by Elisabet Anderson

"Newly Hatched Chick" Page 52 by Brandi Lyn Taylor

"The Sound of Silence" of son, Tom Fouts, Page 65 by Suzanne Fouts

"Biking on the Beach" with Stephanie and Kira Rose Tavill page 74 by Olivia Tavill

"Team Andy" pages 78 and 83 by Mary Lou Stebbins

All other photos by the author.

Table of Contents

DEDICATION Meet Adalyn & Tenley 5

INTRODUCTION 7

CHAPTER ONE Let's start at the very beginning 13

CHAPTER TWO The Decision 21

CHAPTER THREE A Tale of Two Surgeries 29

CHAPTER FOUR A Tale of Two Activations 37

CHAPTER FIVE Auditory Rehab 43

CHAPTER SIX Sounds 49
    "I didn't know butterfly wings made a sound"

CHAPTER SEVEN From There to Hear, ... 57
    From Here to There & From There to Here

CHAPTER EIGHT And Then There's the Rough Spots 63

CHAPTER NINE Other Perspectives 71

CHAPTER TEN Is a Hearing Dog for You? 79
    By Margaret Gerhard

ACKNOWLEDGEMENTS 85

GLOSSARY A Few Definitions 91

ADDITIONAL RESOURCES 92
From Cochlear Implant Basics, by Richard Pocker

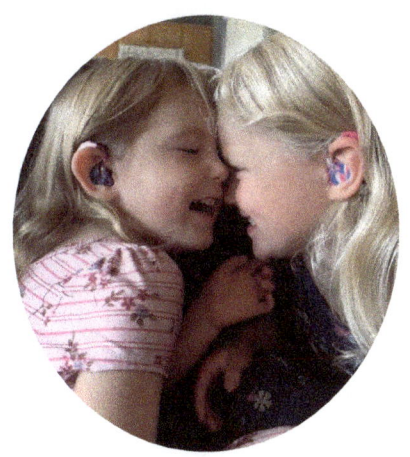

Dedication

I'm dedicating this book to two of my great-great nieces, Tenley on the left, Adalyn on the right.

Adalyn, 8, got her first hearing aids in September 2019, just a few months after my first implant, and Tenley, 6, got hers in April 2020. Both of their hearing losses are bilateral sensorineural hearing loss due to the recessive MYO15A gene (which is non-syndromic). Tenley's loss is mild-severe with severe loss in the high frequencies. Adalyn's loss is severe-profound with the loss being across all frequencies. As of this writing, Adalyn is being evaluated yearly to see if a cochlear implant would be of benefit.

I am so grateful that early detection is now happening and both girls' hearing loss was caught early. I'm also grateful for the progress made in treating hearing loss with state-of-the art hearing aids and/or cochear implants. Tenley and Adalyn truly rock wearing hearing aids and are such great role models for not letting anything stop them from achieving their goals! Currently Adalyn excels at gymnastics and Tenley often scores goals for her soccer team. Not to mention both are excellent students and artists! Watch out world!

Introduction

Let me introduce you to the story about my personal journey into the world of sound with two cochlear implants, and give you a bit of a heads-up as to what's in the following pages.

Success:

First off, it's a success story—about a low-income elderly woman (me), who was living in a remote, rural area in Michigan's Upper Peninsula (UP), and who was gradually going deaf. It's a story about how my progressive sensorineural hearing loss was causing me to isolate. It's a story of how, with two cochlear implants, I have rejoined the world.

It's a story of thousands of miles driven, in all seasons, from my home to a big city in Lower Michigan. It's a story of choosing my team and of how I've been able to add to the team, which as been a win-win for all!

It is also the story of the vital role a supportive community plays. It's about the role of curiosity, and of being able to laugh *and* cry. It's about always keeping an open mind and spirit.

It's a story of perseverance. It's a story of recovery from two surgeries followed by many hours of hard work over a span of weeks, months, years, the work to train my brain to understand the robotic sounds of the implant and translate them into understandable words, music, and environmental sounds. Learning never stops—I'm still hearing new sounds and usually have to ask someone else to tell me what it is that I'm hearing. Or keep playing the "You're hot," "You're cold" game to locate and identify the sound. Oh, and by the way… words and sounds are no longer robotic!

It's an exciting adventure. It's an exhausting adventure. Trust me, when I say *Hearing Fatigue is Real.*

My reason for writing this book is to get information out about cochlear implants. I also want to give hope to older adults who no longer benefit from hearing aid(s). If you are on the fence about getting a cochlear implant, I urge you to do the research, find a cochlear team and see if you qualify, and consider if you are prepared to do the needed auditory rehab work. Your current audiologist can most likely refer you to a cochlear team; if not, contact information for the three cochlear companies is listed in the "Resources Chapter."

I also hope to debunk the myth that only the young benefit from a cochlear implant; that it's too expensive; that it's too far to travel. I live in Michigan's Upper Peninsula, and many places are far to travel. Visits to my Marquette audiologist entailed a 200-mile round trip. Appointments with the cochlear surgeon and audiologist required many 700-mile round trips. It was all so worth it!

Introduction

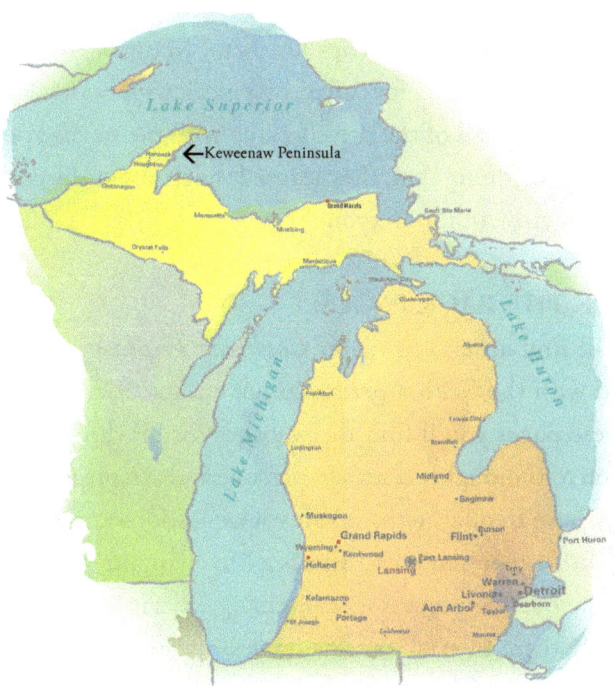

    I obtained my first implant at the age of 76 and the second at the age of 78. There are many people older than me getting a new lease on life thanks to a cochlear implant.

    My cochlear team, and my support system of friends and family, were key! I had to ask for and accept help.

    I stayed with my daughter in Holland, MI and all appointments were in busy Grand Rapids, a half hour to 45 minutes away. I live in a rural area without much traffic and I was not comfortable making the short drive to a large city with fast-moving traffic. Not all appointments coincided with Beth's work schedule. Therefore, I enlisted the help of family and friends, who gladly picked me up at Beth's and drove me to my appointments. Some of the good samaritans lived in Grand Rapids, which entailed two round trips for them. Many of these excursions included stopping for coffee, or a meal, which added a huge social plus. Also all of the drivers came with me to the appointments and, by doing that, they learned much about the cochlear process, a win/win for everyone.

CHECK THE BACK PAGES:
You will find an excerpt from *Cochlear Implant Basics*, reprinted with the written permission of author, Richard Pocker. On these pages you'll find the websites for all three brands. I urge you to thoroughly research each one and after reading about all they have to offer, write down your questions and request to speak with a representative. This is a life-changing decision and while the outside processors can change, what is implanted is hopefully there to stay. Outside processors are only compatible with the brand of the actual implant.

THREE BRANDS: As of this writing, there are three brands of cochlear implants, Cochlear Americas, Med-El, and Advanced Bionics. Each have different options within their product lines. Because I have the Cochlear Americas brand and currently use the N7 processor, that's what I've written about. I chose the Cochlear Americas brand because, not only were reviews excellent, but at the time they were the company that offered Bluetooth connection. Below is a link which, as of this writing, offers a Cochlear Implant Comparison Chart for the three current companies.

https://cochlearimplanthelp.files.wordpress.com/

Introduction

Richard Pocker has also listed some great tips, as well as some key cochlear Facebook pages, in the resources pages in the back of this book, where current users and people exploring getting an implant can connect, ask questions, and share stories.

I'm so pleased that at almost 81 years of age, I can hear and understand the spoken word and many sounds. I am once again involved in the world at large!

I hope you enjoy this book. I'd love to hear from you. Please feel free to email me at there2hear81@gmail.com and check out my new Facebook page From There to Hear.

Carol Rose

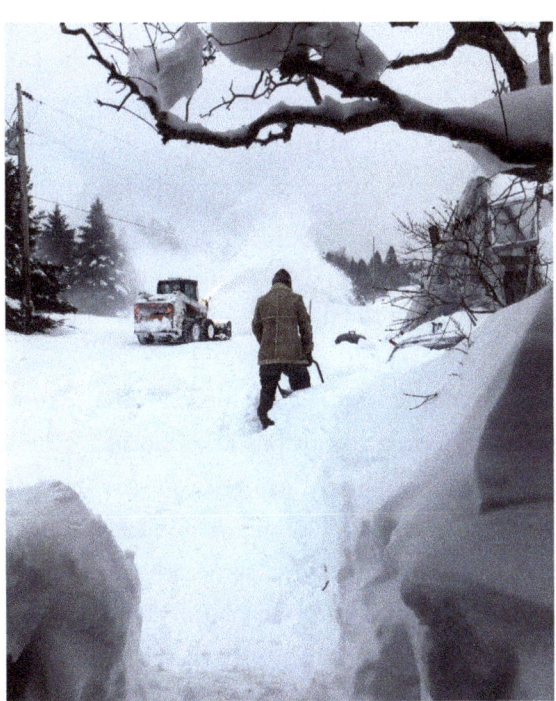

Friends removing snow so I could quickly leave between blizzards for another downstate appointment.

FROM THERE TO HEAR

Hearing Aids and Cochlear Implants
What is the difference?

A cochlear implant is very different than a hearing aid!

Hearing aids amplify sounds so they may be detected by damaged ears. Hearing aids served me well until my hearing loss progressed to the point where they were no longer a benefit.

Cochlear implants bypass damaged portions of the ear and directly stimulate the auditory nerve.

A cochlear implant is a complex medical device providing the sense of sound by electrical stimulation of the auditory nerve directly. They are not a cure and do not restore hearing but provide an opportunity for the person to *perceive* the sensation of sound by bypassing the damaged inner ear. They do not give normal hearing.

As the name implies, cochlear implants require surgery. While I've opted to not put any photos of the incision, required stitches, scars, etc., I can tell you that in my case, the incision was about four inches long, behind and above my ear. While my surgeon used stitches, some others use glue, tape, or staples. I had about an inch or two of hair shaved, (which grew back), and the remaining small scar is barely visible.

CHAPTER ONE
Let's Start at the Very Beginning

☙

"Let's start at the very beginning, a very good place to start." That's what Julie Andrews sang in *The **Sound** of Music*. And since I'm talking about "**Sound**," and often asked how my hearing loss came about—when and the cause—I thought it would be good if I started with the very beginning.

I was born in 1942 and there were no hearing tests back then. Not in the hospital (or home, as that is where I made my entrance). Nor in the schools…there were no preschool physical checkups. There was no "preschool"—it was kindergarten and then on to elementary and high school. I don't remember ever having my hearing checked.

Because I had frequent earaches, I had my ears checked by the family doctor, but I'm sure even he did not concern himself with a possible hearing loss.

Looking at my childhood and teen years, I'm sure I always (or since I was very young) have had some level of hearing loss. It was not substantial, as I don't have the speech pattern that could be caused by a significant hearing loss. However, I mispronounce a good deal of words, due most likely to never hearing them correctly. Recently I told a niece

I was going to pick up some "rosatierre chicken." She kindly let me know it was called "rotisserie chicken." Between having dyslexia and hearing loss, *rosatierre* was my word of choice. Now, I need to stop and think before I say that word. Speech therapy!

In school, I thought I was dumb, stupid, as I simply could not get assignments correct. Now I believe I just did not understand the teacher. I understood enough to just get by.

I worked in a dry cleaners starting at age 14, tagging clothes and waiting on customers. I don't remember having an issue there.

However, when I went to work at a very busy grocery store in my senior year of high school, I did not do well at all. With my current knowledge of hearing loss, I'm confident it was partially due to the extreme noise and my inability to understand directions and customers.

In early adulthood, I was employed as a clerk/secretary at Brunswick Corporation, and I made a huge mistake in copying some papers, which cost the company money in the form of my wages, paper and ink. It was the early 60s and copying was via a mimeograph machine. I printed hundreds of pages before my supervisor saw my mistake. I believe my error was in misunderstanding the verbal instructions.

I didn't realize I had a hearing loss until I was in my 30s. My husband and I were fostering a child with developmental disabilities. I don't know how I knew but I just knew that in addition to his mental and learning disabilities, he was also hard of hearing. I made an appointment for him with Marlene Bevan, Audiologist and owner of Audiocare Hearing Center in Traverse

Chapter 1: Let's Start at the Very Beginning

City, Michigan. While there, she said to me, "Carol, when is the last time you had *your* hearing tested?"

"I've never had it tested," I replied. I'm not sure what it was she saw or heard at that moment, which made her suspicious of a possible hearing loss. Perhaps I misunderstood her, asked her to repeat herself, needed to look at her or my foster son's face to lip read, or maybe talked very loud. All signs of possible hearing loss. Whatever it was that alerted her, she set me up for an appointment. Sure enough, her suspicions were correct. I had a moderate sensorineural hearing loss (SNHL) in both ears.

No Solution

It was the early 1970s and at that time there was no hearing aid available for my particular hearing loss. So, I did what I had been doing for so many years, without even realizing that I was doing it. I did what so many hard of hearing people do, I continued using various coping mechanisms. I smiled when I couldn't hear at gatherings, or I just backed away from conversations. I stayed away from group discussions. And I got into arguments with my spouse as I would misunderstand what he was saying. We tried, mostly unsuccessfully, using the tactic of me saying "Did I hear you say…?" I mention this here as it is so very common among so many couples where one has a hearing loss. When hearing declines, relationships are affected and often the person who is hard of hearing is reluctant to be told that they are not hearing well, so broaching the subject can be difficult. Studies show that treatment of hearing loss, via hearing aids or surgery, results in significant improvements in relationships.

FROM THERE TO HEAR

I was living in Traverse City, Michigan when I found out I had a hearing loss and since there was nothing that could be done at that time, I just continued to live life as best I could, with four young kids and a couple of special needs foster kids.

My family would often get irritated with me when I would ask "what?" or when I would completely misunderstand their words. The kids learned early on to say, "But I told you, you just didn't hear me," when confronted about not letting me know about something. They admitted in their adult years that they had often used this as an excuse, knowing I could not refute it.

When a second testing a short time later showed additional hearing loss, the audiologist referred me to the University of Michigan. I went there at least once a year for a battery of tests to try to determine the cause. The results always came back "progressive SNHL, etiology (*the cause*) unknown." However, hearing aid companies kept developing new technology and eventually there were aids that would help me. Unfortunately, this was not before I had to turn down a coveted job offer.

I was working at the Traverse City Record Eagle sometime in the late 1970s/early 1980s. I started out in the "tape room," going to work in the wee hours of the morning and sorting the Associated Press tapes into working order for the editors to look at when they arrived. I enjoyed the whole atmosphere of the newspaper. It didn't matter what I was doing, I was part of the magic of this printed paper getting out every single day! I also worked in the "morgue," making sense of the old articles and categorizing them for the reporters to have easy access.

Note: this was all before computers! I began doing some reporting. Then one day when reporter Mike Norton said loudly,

Chapter 1: Let's Start at the Very Beginning

"I'm done with the church pages!," I volunteered to take them over. I loved it; I could do the interviews as they were one-on-one, and I could understand the other person if we were in a quiet setting.

Note: the newsroom itself was NOT a quiet setting! There was a constant clacking of typewriters. Some were old standard uprights, some modern electric, but still noisy, and there were no cubicles. It was one very large newsroom and at deadline especially, reporters and editors did not bother to leave their typewriters to ask or answer a question; they would shout out over the constant hum of the typewriters and conversation. However, there was always a quiet room I could use to interview someone. I absolutely loved it there.

Then came the day I had been waiting for. A full-time reporter's position opened and was offered to me. However, all reporters took turns covering local meetings…school boards, township, county, etc. This was before hearing aids were appropriate for my hearing loss. I knew, because of my hearing loss, I would not be able to hear and understand at the noisy meetings. I could have taped some of the meeting, but that wouldn't have caught the needed comments from the audience. I turned down the offer. Both the Managing Editor, Mike Ready, and I were in tears. I have written all my life and I pined for this position. Reflecting on this passionate and deep disappointment, I believe writing may well have been a coping mechanism for my hearing loss, which I didn't know had.

The American with Disabilities Act (ADA) was not passed until 1990, but even if it had been in effect, there was little in the way of assistive technology available for the hard of hearing.

I turned in my resignation that day. I would no longer be content to do the small reporting job. While I had built the religion page up to three pages of stories, I was bored with it, and it needed someone with new ideas.

I did however, create a job for myself. The paper was putting out something called "Summer Pages," a tabloid featuring the tourist towns around Traverse City. There were three of us on this "made to order" team. Harry was the photographer and there was a salesperson from the ad department. I would interview *(again one-to-one, which I could still do)*, and write about businesses, residents and tourists. It was a great summer freelance job and I proved to myself that I could earn a living from my writing.

New Technology

Somewhere in the early 1980s I was finally able to be fitted with hearing aids, which helped tremendously. Eventually, other assistive devices were also made available. There were amplifiers for phones, external microphones, alarm systems and more. Things were improving for the hard of hearing. When I moved to Michigan's Upper Peninsula (UP) in 1995/96, I volunteered for the Hearing Loss of America Michigan Chapter as a Hearing Technology Resource Specialist (HTRS), a rewarding and enjoyable position. Technology was moving fast, and many improvements were made. The HTRS team demonstrated the new assistive technology devices to hard of hearing groups, audiologists, retirement centers and more.

Chapter 1: Let's Start at the Very Beginning

Peepers (Spring Frogs)

It was Spring of 2001. I was wearing Phonak hearing aids, which had a wireless Bluetooth microphone, allowing me to hear conversations in noisy situations. It also allowed a friend to introduce me to spring peepers *(tiny frogs, which make a loud sound)*. I grew up near lakes, rivers and creeks; we called them "cricks" back then—or at least I think that is what we called them. I guess I better ask someone!

There had to be peepers—yet I had never heard the sound before. On our family vacations my husband would go outside at night to listen to the frogs. I know now he was hearing the magical singing of the peepers. Back then I had no clue. I only knew frogs made the deep throaty "rebbit" sound. The day my friend introduced me to the peepers' mating song was pure magic. We were riding together next to a lake in the UP and he said "Wow, listen to the peepers." I had no clue what he was talking about. He took my microphone, which was connected via Bluetooth to my hearing aids, and went down to the lake. Had I been by myself, I would have sworn we were being attacked from outer space.

Because of the technological advancements, I was able to continue to partake in family and community events. However, my hearing loss was progressive. Eventually, even state-of-the-art hearing aids and assistive technology such as wireless microphones, did not work. This led me to explore the possibility of getting cochlear implants.

Here's a fun note from a great-niece, Chelsea, *(mom of Adalyn and Tenley, who are featured on the Dedication Page)* regarding my wireless microphone: "I remember thinking the microphone was magic when I could talk to you from another room. So thankful for this technology."

NOTE: When it comes to hearing loss, there are three main types: sensorineural, conductive and mixed. An audiologist can help you determine the degree of your loss, a possible cause, and will help find solutions, which might be hearing aids or other assistive devices, or a possible referral to a specialist.

CHAPTER TWO
The Decision

Fast Forward to 2017

- I had given up doing interviews for my newspaper reporting job because I no longer understood the person I was interviewing.
- I stopped attending public events—not even for fun, as I could no longer get by with nodding and smiling.
- I stopped making and accepting phone calls unless someone was present to help interpret as I could not understand the other person on the phone.
- I declined invites to events with more than one other person, as I could not keep up with conversations.
- I had some special microphones and other equipment, which previously made understanding conversations over the phone and in noise "do-able." This was no longer the case.
- **I was isolating.** I knew from my research that hearing loss was a possible risk factor for dementia and that isolation was a main cause.*

*See study by Frank Lin, MD, PhD, of Johns Hopkins University on page 27.

September 2017

I attended a family event—a wedding in fact—one where I presided over the marriage of a grandson and his wife.

Even though there were many people invited, I was sure I'd be ok, because it was outside. The ceremony was went smoothly as it was just Mike, Jen and me speaking. However, afterwards there were many different conversations happening at once. The fact that there was intermittent rain, and we all had to gather under a tent, made understanding conversations next to impossible. Even when the rain cleared and we were outside, where there was lots of space, background noise of music and many people talking, made it impossible to understand what people were saying, unless I was off to the side talking one-to-one.

I felt lost…left out…not because of anything anyone did or said—especially not because of what anyone said, because, for the most part I had no clue what they said. It was all mumbles. I also knew they were not mumbling. However, what I heard was merely mumbles.

NOTE: One of the first clues that someone has a hearing loss—they say "people mumble"—when they most likely are not mumbling

Could my increased hearing loss be something simple?
Perhaps the issue was caused by wax in my ears. Maybe both hearing aids had deteriorated. In my heart I knew both these theories were most unlikely.

Chapter 2: The Decision

December 2017

I made an appointment with my audiologist, **Jackie Gilbert**, MS, CCC-A of Superior Ear, Nose & Throat Specialists in Marquette, Michigan.

While in the booth listening to sounds and words, I knew I was failing this test. When I came out Jackie said, "Carol, you know we have discussed possibilities when hearing aids and assistive devices no longer work for you..." I knew what we had discussed. The possibility of getting a cochlear implant—maybe two.

I did not want surgery!

I cried...Jackie comforted me. I took a deep breath in and said "Ok, what's next?"

Together we decided to try new "state of the art hearing aids." I applaud Jackie for letting me give hearing aids another whirl. It took a while to order, receive and program the new aids.

2018

The first "public event" I attended with these new hearing aids was a family winter weekend at the Porcupine Mountains, located in the Western part of Michigan's Upper Peninsula.

I went. I snowshoed and I tried to play board games and I attempted to converse with the others. Outside in the quiet of the woods, I could understand the person who was right next to me, as long as they took time to look at me so I could see their lips. This was not the case with those who were ahead or behind. And definitely not the case inside the noisy cabin.

It felt like my whole family had learned a foreign language and forgot to tell me.

I went home from that weekend sad and scared. I knew the new aids were not the answer but I did not want someone cutting into my head.

Shortly thereafter I received a notice of the 2018 Hearing Loss Association of America, Michigan State Association's Annual Meeting, which was to be held in Lansing on April 21. The featured speaker was Dr. Kara Leyzac, from the Kresge Hearing Research Institute, who would be discussing research updates, (including Cochlear Implants). I asked my daughter, Beth, who lived fairly close to the meeting location, if she would like to go with me. She did.

Dr. Leyzac was inspiring—***but*** it was a lunchtime conversation with a friend that clinched my decision to pursue an implant. I had known Juanita for more than 25 years and we had worked together as Hearing Technology Resource Specialists, (HRTRS). We shared a similar history of progressive hearing loss, and both of us had talked about how much we did not want surgery!

However, since I had last seen her, she had received two cochlear implants. Her ability to converse with us in a noisy room and especially her response to a question aimed at her back was heartening to both Beth and me.

"Nice meeting you," Beth said to Juanita as she walked away, and was shocked when Juanita turned around and said, "Nice meeting you too."

"Mom, she could not see my face, and she understood me!"

I went back to Jackie, my audiologist, and took the next step. Even though I was receiving Social Security, and freelancing for a newspaper, I was still in the "low-income" category. So, if I was approved for the implant procedure, Medicare and Medicaid would cover most, if not all the expenses.

Choosing a Cochlear Team

Jackie usually referred her patients to the cochlear team at the University of Michigan (U of M). However, I wanted to go to a place closer to my daughter's town of Holland, MI, as I would need support and a place to stay.

My community of family and friends, both near and far, played such an important, wonderful role throughout the entire process of getting not only one but two cochlear implants

Jackie's contact at U of M suggested I try to get into ENT Specialist/Surgeon Dr. Robert Daniels, of ENT Center in Grand Rapids. It took a some time, (including getting referral letters from Jackie and Dr. David Heichel, MD, of Superior ENT Specialists in Marquette, MI, as well as many phone calls). I finally succeeded in getting an appointment with Dr. Daniels and then with Dr. Darcy Jaarsma, AuD, CCC-A, the audiologist at Spectrum Health, (now Corewell Health) with whom he worked.

Once I made the decision to move forward and begin exploring the qualifying process to see if I was a candidate for cochlear implants, I experienced no fear—until activation day—which you will read about later in this book.

My reason for writing this book is to get information out about cochlear implants. I also want to give hope to older adults who no longer benefit from hearing aid(s). If you are on the fence about getting a cochlear implant, I urge you to do the research, find a cochlear team and see if you qualify. Your current audiologist can most likely refer you to a cochlear team; if not, contact information for the three cochlear companies is listed in the "Resources Chapter."

If the exams by the surgeon and cochlear audiologist determine that you do qualify, the surgeon's office and the cochlear company you choose will help you get pre-approved by your insurance company. If your insurance company denies coverage, your surgeon's office and the company representatives can help with resubmitting. It could be as simple as a incorrect code. Persistence is key. In my case, Medicare/Medicaid paid 100% of my surgeries and post-op appointments with the surgeon and audiologist. It also covered my external processors and some assistive technology devices. I only had very small co-pay for post-op prescription meds. I live in Michigan, and because of my low-income status, I received Medical Mileage reimbursement through the state's Department of Human Services. I had the choice of having a state certified driver take me to my appointments or driving myself. I filed the necessary paperwork regarding my capability and was my own "designated driver."

Because I was low-income employed and needed technical assistance to keep my job as a writer/reporter/ad salesperson, Michigan Department of Vocational Rehab paid for a new hearing aid for my non-implanted side, which was compatible with the Cochlear Americas processor I chose. They also paid for an iPhone and a laptop, both which I could stream to the new processor and hearing aid.

Note: A person's hearing, with hearing aids, needs to be low enough to meet the current and ever-changing cochlear

Chapter 2: The Decision

implant criteria. Expanding criteria has made cochlear implants an option for many more people, not only the severely hearing impaired. Because changes are happening rapidly, please check with your audiologist to get the most recently qualifying criteria. An audiologist, who has training in cochlear implants, is a necessary team player.

Also, a person's primary physician needs to clear them for surgery. My cochlear surgeon gave a specific list of medical tests required prior to surgery, which included an-MRI.

New Study Links Hearing Loss with Dementia in Older Adults Published January 2023

I've been following the research that connects dementia with hearing loss for several years. In fact, it was one of the leading concerns I had when realizing hearing aids were no longer meeting my needs and I found myself isolating.

Earlier research conducted by Frank Lin, MD, PhD of John Hopkins University, showed some of the possible causes of the link between hearing loss and dementia to be:

- "People with hearing loss tend to feel isolated, since it's hard to join in conversations or be social with others when you can't hear. Some research has shown a link between feeling lonely or isolated and dementia. So hearing loss may make mental decline happen faster than it would otherwise.
- ""If your ears can no longer pick up on as many sounds, your hearing nerves will send fewer signals to your brain. As a result, the brain declines."

"It's likely a combination of all three," says Lin, who has done much of the research on the connection between the conditions.

The January 2023 publication was based on further studies involving more than 2,400 older adults and were found to be consistent with prior studies showing that hearing loss might be a contributing factor to dementia risk over time, and that treating hearing loss may lower dementia risk.

More information can be found at:
https://publichealth.jhu.edu/2023/new-study-links-hearing-loss-with-dementia-in-older-adults

CHAPTER THREE
A Tale of Two Surgeries
1-10-19 at age 76 and 3-25-21 at age 78

☙☙

What is cochlear implant surgery?

Surgery consists of an incision behind and, as in my case, sometimes a bit above the ear. An opening is created in the mastoid bone and the electrodes are guided through and placed inside the cochlea. A pocket is made between the muscle and bone behind the ear for an internal processor and magnet. The magnet then connects to the external processor. The surgery is usually done under general anesthesia and generally takes between two and three hours. Most surgeries are done on an out patient basis.

The patient does not hear immediately following surgery. Hearing does not occur until the external sound processor is attached to the patient's head; its magnet connecting with the magnet inside the skull. The cochlear audiologist will activate the implant using a computer program. Although some clinics are now scheduling activation for the day following surgery, this usually happens two to six weeks after surgery, when the swelling has gone down and healing has taken place. More about activation in the next chapter.

My Tale of Two Surgeries:

I've written about the process of losing my hearing, and the decision to explore cochlear implants. And then there's the actual surgery, which I had been so against having. Now, four years post the first implant and two years post the second, I do 'daily gratefuls' for everything I can hear and understand! **I never have a single regret!**

Surgery #1; January 10, 2019

Once I made my up mind to move forward, there was no fear of the upcoming surgery. Only excitement, even as I was being wheeled into the operating room. However, in the first 48 hours following surgery, I was NOT convinced I had done the right thing.

Surgery, which was planned as a mid-morning outpatient process, ended up being pushed back to mid-afternoon and included an overnight stay as I was so very dizzy, nauseous and in severe pain. Because there were no overnight plans in place, an empty bed was found, but on a surgical floor where patients had experienced some sort of gastrointestinal surgery. When the shift changed, the new nurse walked in, started looking for my chart and asked how my stomach was. "She had head surgery," dead-panned my daughter, Beth. The nurse then looked up and, with a rather sheepish look on his face, saw the bandages wrapped around my head.

Despite that little glitch, I was well taken care of and had some control over the IV pain meds. I was given ice packs and anti-nausea meds. Beth was recovering from shoulder surgery herself and was also given ice packs. Special treatment for

Chapter 3: A Tale of Two Surgeries

my special caregiver. By mid-morning of the following day, I was well enough to get dressed and was on my way to Beth's house to continue the recovery process.

POST SURGERY BRAIN FOG: By late in the day, I felt well enough to venture to the kitchen and even visit briefly with a friend. However, the next morning when Beth came in to check on me, she was surprised at my report of being in a LOT of pain and so very nauseous. I had my meds beside my bed and had faithfully taken them during the night and even logged what I took and when. Hah! I had faithfully taken the WRONG meds. In my post-surgery brain fog, I had taken the antibiotics instead of the pain pills. I write about this as we learned how important it is to have someone other than the patient in charge of the meds for the first couple days, while the anesthesia is still so very active and messing with the thinking process.

PUSHING THE ENVELOPE: I was working for a local newspaper and a few days after surgery, I was at the computer writing and editing other's writings, and also working on ads. This was with extremely blurry vision and an equally dizzy head. Not smart! I also opted to make the 377-mile trip from Beth's home in Holland, Michigan to my home in Grand Marais, MI on January 18, as soon as I got the go-ahead from the surgeon the day before saying I that could drive. This was doubly not smart! Fortunately, I took two days to make the drive, stopping to rest for a night.

I was pushing the envelope and, while going back to work so soon, and making the numerous long drives back and forth for needed appointments had no detrimental consequences to my hearing journey, I know it slowed my physical healing/

recovery process. In order to heal, a body needs to rest, and while this is important to all ages, I know this need increases with age.

SUCCESS: Some of the side effects from surgery #1, included dizziness, some loss of balance, and a wayward electrode causing some pain. Not only did all of these eventually lessen or dissipate, they were overridden by the awesomeness of being able to rejoin the world; to experience not only hearing and understanding the spoken word, but sounds, some of which I had never heard…oh and music!

NOTE: This awesome outcome only came after **activation** and hours and hours of **auditory rehab**. Therefore, in 2020, when my audiologist informed me that Medicare/Medicaid would now cover a second implant, I readily began the process again. This time around was much easier as I already had my cochlear team and I knew the drill. I quickly set up appointments with my surgeon, cochlear audiologist and primary physician.

Surgery #2; March 25, 2021

When I was cleared by the surgeon to have the second implant, I asked Beth if she was ready to be my support person again. "Only if you agree to stay with me from the surgery to the activation, and not make the long trips back and forth so soon after surgery."

Some cochlear implant recipients resume regular, non-athletic, with no lifting activities, a week to 10 days after surgery. Most likely they are not 76 (first surgery) or 78 (second surgery) years old. While, people older than me successfully have cochlear implants, I am also aware that my body simply does not heal as fast as it did 10, 20 or more years ago. It's important to know yourself and your personal limits and levels of tolerance!

Not only did I agree to Beth's stipulations, my friend, Len, agreed to stay with my cat and dog, **and** I took six weeks off from the newspaper.

Two Surgeries, Two Different Results

The surgeon now administered prednisone during surgery and a 10-day tapering supply after. I also received anti-nausea meds pre, during and post surgery, as well as a prescription for pain meds. Staying longer at my daughter's and these tweaks made this second surgery so much easier than the first.

NOTE: When, during my pre-op appointment for the second implant, Dr. Daniels told me that he now gave the prednisone, I politely, but firmly told him "No thank you," He wanted to know why I was declining. I explained that I was not interested in having the after-effects I had heard about from people taking prednisone. He explained that not only would the medication help reduce swelling and inflammation but would also help with the healing process. He assured me that the side effects would be minimal as, following surgery, I would be on a 10-day tapering schedule. He let me know I might have increased appetite and some mild anxiety. After hearing that, and trusting his knowledge and skills, I agreed. While I didn't notice any increase in appetite, when I had two meltdowns a few days after surgery over very minor happenings, Beth said "Mom, what *IS* going on?" With that question, I remembered Dr. Daniels' mentioning the possibility of some anxiety . Beth and my granddaughter, Mena, and I began questioning if I should stay on the prednisone. While Beth was contacting the pharmacy for info, I was searching on-line. The pharmacist advised to continue the medication and I also found facts supporting its use with cochlear implant surgery. The three of us decided we could all handle any meltdowns as we now knew what was causing them and knew it would be short term.

    HEALING: I let myself relax and heal. I began walking inside and then around Beth's subdivision; short, slow walks and staying close to her house in the beginning, in case dizziness occurred. I gradually increased my walking boundaries.

    By the time I left for home, I was very physically recovered, walking three to five miles a day.

    The second surgery took place early in the morning. And by mid-afternoon I was feeling good and on my way to Beth's. As you can see by the picture (below) the coil and magnet were under the bandage and were connected via the magnet to my first implant. The processor was taped to the bandage, allowing me to hear as soon as I woke up in the recovery room.

    Shortly after arriving at her house, the processor beeped, signaling me that the battery needed to be changed.

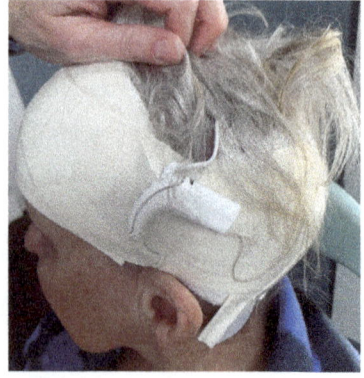
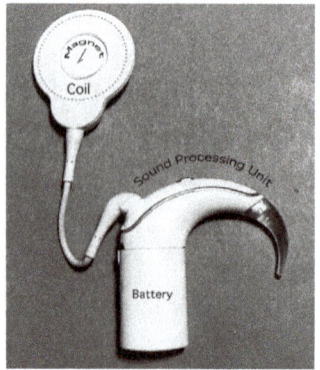

N7 Processor

Chapter 3: A Tale of Two Surgeries

Silence, Stone Cold Deaf Silence

I knew I'd be deaf.
I was ready to be deaf, or so I thought.
Deaf—total deafness!
Reality hit hard as my daughter changed the battery of my first processor, which was taped to the outside of the bandages encompassing my head.
With the battery off, I began to talk, only to realize I could not hear my own voice!
I didn't know—hadn't realized—what total deafness meant.
Reality hit—hit hard. I could not hear myself speak.
I had no voice!
Sobs shook my body as reality of the new sound of silence hit.
The battery replaced, I tried to tell her what had happened; tried to tell her about not hearing myself. We held each other. We both wept.
We both took deep breaths.
"Feel your throat Mom, feel your throat."
Vibrations!
Vibrations indicating that even if I couldn't hear my voice, it was still there.
There in the sounds of silence!

FROM THERE TO HEAR

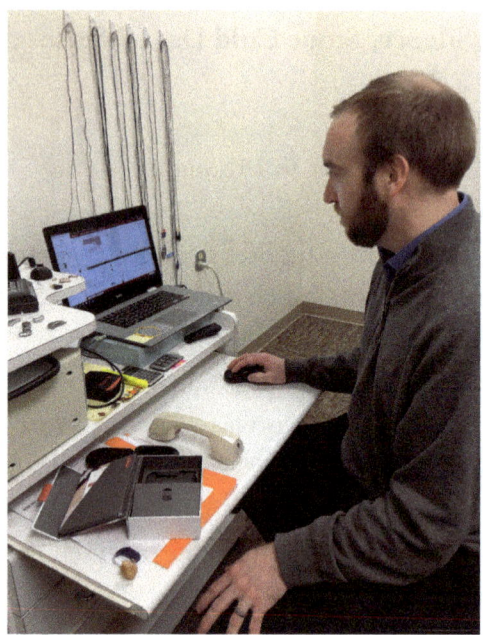

With my first cochlear implant it was important to get a hearing aid for my other ear, which would be compatible with my Cochlear Nucleus 7 Processor. With the financial help of Michigan Rehabilitation Services and the technical help of Audiologist, Brian Kuopus of Superior Hearing in Marquette, MI, this need was met. Brian ordered and programmed the ReSound Hearing aid. At my first activation, Darcy Jaarsma, my cochlear audiologist at Spectrum Hospital in Grand Rapids, MI paired it to my new processor so both would automatically connect via Bluetooth to my iPhone.

CHAPTER FOUR
A Tale of Two Activations

❦

What is Activation?

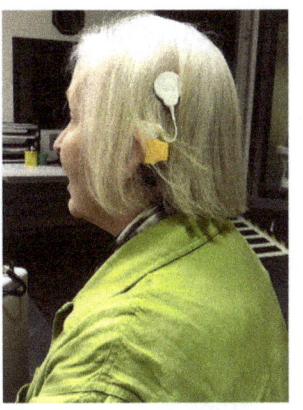

"At an initial activation, the audiologist sets the amount of stimulation required for the patient to "hear" sound with the implant. In the beginning, the recipient may not be able to tolerate very much stimulation, so that's why we create progressively "louder" programs that the recipient can work up to as they get used to hearing with the implant. At subsequent appointments, the "map" is fine tuned to provide the best possible sound quality to the recipient (think graphic equalizer on a stereo—the audiologist can adjust the stimulation of the various electrodes to optimize the sound for the recipient).

by Dr . Darcy Jaarsma

February 19, 2019
Meeting Jeremiah: *Activation of First Implant*

I want to tell you how I felt when I woke up on Monday, February 18, 2019. It was five and a half weeks after my first cochlear surgery, the day of the scheduled "activation" of my first implant. The day I would hear something. Or would I? I was overcome with FEAR! Intense FEAR! FEAR I would hear NOTHING! I shared this with a couple friends, and they listened and walked/talked/drummed and wrote me through it. By late morning, I was more confident, happy and ready to roll.

However, there must have been some fear remaining, witnessed my intense reaction on two videos taken by my daughter, Beth, which showed how relieved I was when I heard the first sound.

My cochlear audiologist, Dr. Darcy Jaarsma, had connected my new processor to her computer (via the yellow item in the photo on the previous page) and the processor's magnet was placed over the magnet inside my head.

This allowed the processor, which rested on my ear, to communicate with the receiver/stimulator inside my head, sending different sound waves through an electrode array, which ran through my mastoid bone and wrapped around my cochlea, sending stimulation to my auditory nerve.

There were no words, just sounds, as Darcy tested the electrodes and found all 22 working! I was thrilled to know I could hear the sounds!

When I heard her voice (even though I could not understand the words—except when reading her lips) and then heard my own voice—I giggled—I laughed—I cried tears of joy! It sounded like ET or the Chipmunks on high-speed. Or like when you inhale air from a helium balloon or play a 75-rpm record at 45-rpm speed (or is it vice versa?). There was a few seconds delay between speaking and hearing my voice.

I named the robot inside my head Jeremiah as I could not "understand a single word he said."

"Jeremiah was a bullfrog
Was a good friend of mine
I never understood a single word he said
But I helped him a-drink his wine
And he always had some mighty fine wine"

I went back to Beth's and immediately began the prescribed auditory rehab process.

Journal entry: Saturday, February 23, 2019

And here I am five days after activation—hearing and understanding more each day. I'm working hard at it with programs on my iPhone, listening to audio books, reading the printed copy while listening; reading out loud what I type, talking to myself…it's rather exhausting. Last night I was in bed at 8pm and didn't rise till 7 this morning. It all still sounds like a robot—but I'm getting to know the robot's language…and I appreciate every step forward.

Fast Forward Two Years To Second Activation Friday, April 15, 2021
Journal entry:

Not only was recovery from the second surgery so very much easier, I had no fear on Activation Day. I was so very pleasantly surprised to be able to hear and understand Dr. Darcy and my daughter at activation. *They were high pitched and tinny to be sure, but I could tell what they were saying.*

Mapping

There's an important process in the cochlear implant world, which takes place at the many post-op audiology appointments. It's called "mapping." The audiologist hooks my processors up to her computer and proceeds to play sounds. I listen carefully letting her know the moment I can detect the tone for each electrode. Through this process she will find my T-levels (thresholds). Then she will find my C-levels (comfort levels) as I give her hand signals as to whether the sound is too loud, too low, or just right. (Kind of like Goldilocks and the Three Bears.) Often, I ask her to go up to where the sound is uncomfortably loud and then decrease it by a dab. This process has remained the same over the past four years, but the frequency of needed to have mappings has decreased to yearly appointments. However, if I notice a change in my ability to understand, or sounds get too quiet, I can make an appointment to be evaluated by my cochlear audiologist before the year is up to see if a new mapping might be needed.

Mapping is the process of programming the cochlear implant. The surgically inserted receiver/stimulator contains many electrodes which are responsible for stimulating different frequencies or pitches. During mapping, the audiologist sets the amount of stimulation required for the individual to perceive sound at a variety of different frequencies (pitches).
By Dr. Darcy Jaarsma

Chapter 4: A Tale of Two Activations

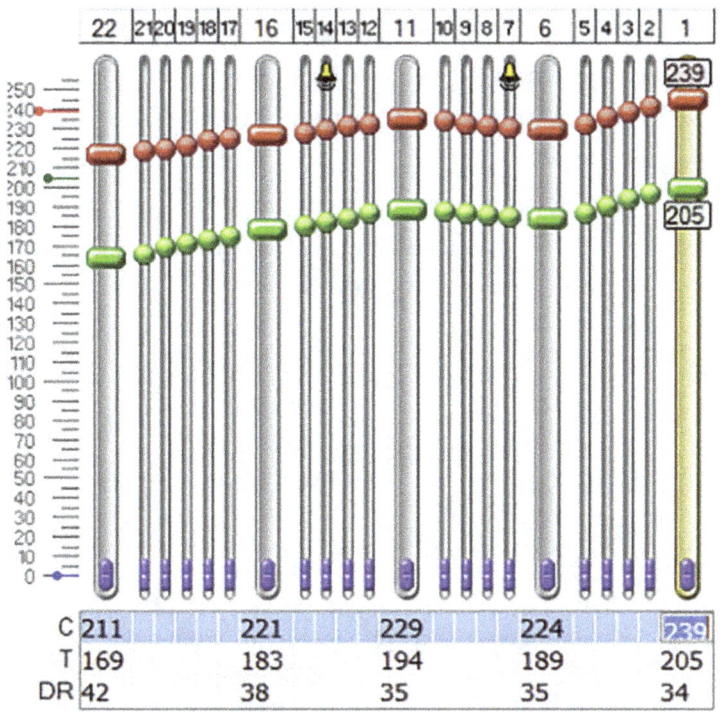

An image of one of my many mappings.

First Mapping Appointment for 2nd Implant
April 23, 2021
Journal Entry

*Here is is, only a week past activation, I had **91% speech recognition** today, in quiet environments/surroundings (no background noise) with only the new processor. It was amazing. It took me about six months to get to this point with the first activation.*

Note on Activation: As with all other aspects of the cochlear implant process, the results are different for everyone. Some only hear beeps and whistles, or perhaps static. Others hear and understand words fairly clear right away. As I experienced, there was a vast difference in my ability to hear and understand the spoken word after the second implant and subsequent activation compared to the first two years earlier.

The one thing that remains consistent is the need for commitment to auditory training.

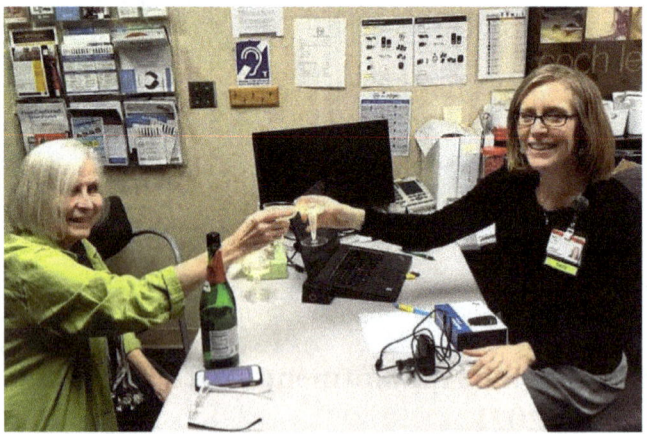

Carol Rose and Audiologist Darcy Jaarsma, toast to a successful 2019 activation with a glass of sparkling grape juice.

CHAPTER FIVE
Auditory Rehab

❧

IMPORTANT:
This might well be the most important chapter in the book because if the person receiving the cochlear implant is not totally committed to doing the auditory rehab work, why get tsurgery? When a person undergoes a joint replacement, they know physical therapy is essential in the recovery process back to normalcy. While a cochlear implant will never replace "normal" hearing, it certainly does give the most recipients the opportunity to be part of society, to hear conversations, music, and environmental sounds, **IF** they do the auditory rehab.

However, I state "most" as this is not always the case, and some people will only ever get environmental sounds, even if they do rehab.

Some of the reasons for varying results are the age the when hearing was lost as well as the length of time between the loss of hearing and the cochlear implant surgery. The possibilities of the degree of success and the part auditory rehab will play in the success, should be discussed with your cochlear team at the pre surgery appointments.

Have you seen "The Sound of Metal"? It's the story of a metal drummer, Ruben, who loses his hearing and gets cochlear implants. If I had seen the movie before getting implanted, I might not have considered this surgery. He ended up ditching the processors and chose to remain in the deaf world. While some people in the deaf community choose not to get cochlear implants, Ruben's story is different. He lost his hearing, got implants but apparently received no advice from his cochlear team about the possible outcome or the need for auditory rehab. He had surgery, was activated and, as many of us do, heard only noise. It appears no one told him, and he didn't do his own research into the needed auditory rehab. The movie won many awards, and I can see why—the acting was superb, but it is so not the reality for most cochlear implant recipients.

One review is here:
https://consumer.hearingreview.com/ sound-of-metal-rings-false-for-cochlear-implant-users/

It is so important for anyone contemplating getting a cochlear implant to commit to the auditory rehab process.

What a Cochlear Implant is NOT:
It is NOT instant hearing! And it's NOT "normal" hearing.

The cochlear processor picks up sound waves, transferring them to the receiver inside my head, which takes them down to the cochlea and on to my brain.

It takes time and training to learn to interpret the signals received from a cochlear implant. While mine certainly sounds "normal" now, I know I'm hearing differently from my typically hearing friends and family. Also, I still lip read. Some cochlear recipients have chosen to let that skill go. I practice hearing without lip reading when riding in a car or walking beside someone. I believe it's still a valuable resource when it comes to communicating in restaurants, groups, etc.

Upon receiving my implant and then getting it activated, it became my task to train my brain to translate these sound waves into words and recognizable everyday sounds, such as the refrigerator, car blinkers, etc.

For my first implant, in 2019, I spent hours each day, for weeks, talking out loud to myself. My audiologist advised me to wear the cochlear processor all day, leaving out my hearing aid, so my brain would be forced to learn the processor's language. I followed her instructions, mostly but I would put the aid in if I was in a situation where I really needed to understand—or when I was just exhausted from the auditory rehab.

I listened to audio books, while reading the printed words of the actual book. I'd go over and over the same sentences, listening and reading, and then would try just listening, until I could make out the spoken words. When I could understand one sentence without reading along, I'd move on to the next. Then to paragraphs, pages, etc. To begin with, even once I could understand them, they still sounded "tinny."

I listened to Ted Talks, using captions at first. I enlisted family and friends to be on the other end of the line and with my phone connected via bluetooth, I began making phone calls, with their voice being streamed direct into my processor. They were very patient as I would ask them to repeat words and/or to go slower. I worked through a variety of auditory rehab programs available on my iPhone.

Auditory Rehab Possible Without Compatible Technology

While my iPhone and computer were extremely helpful for me during my rehab process, it is not necessary to have a compatible phone, tablet, or computer to do auditory rehab. One of my friends had sudden deafness, necessitating two cochlear implants within a short time. He did not have any compatible electronics and learned the implant's language by going out fishing alone and talking to himself, the fish, loons, eagles and other wildlife while he was out there. There are also programs online, which can be printed out for others to read certain words, sentences, paragraphs to you.

It's important to talk to your cochlear audiologist prior to surgery to get their recommendations on what auditory rehab would work best for you. And consider joining one of the Cochlear Facebook groups so you can be in touch with others who are experiencing similar issues.

How Long Will Brain Training Take?

My brain training will continue—forever. I am constantly hearing new environmental sounds, and often have to ask someone what I'm hearing. Sometimes they have to think hard and make themselves pay attention as it might be a comon sound they no longer notice; it has faded into the background for them. Wind was one, as were different bird sounds. I'm also learning new words. I was at a restaurant with a friend and the waitress did not

Chapter 5: Auditory Rehab

have a name tag. My friend asked her name. I could not figure it out. Both my friend and the waitress were patient in repeating it...slowly, until I got it.

My cochlear team, the surgeon, his nurse, and my audiologist, all did a good job of letting me know sounds would not sound "normal" and it would take time and much practice, before they did. Everyone is different. Some people understand words at activation—others not for months. With my first implant's activation, while I could tell words were being spoken, I could not understand them, and they sounded high-pitched and tinny. With my second implant's activation, while they were tinny, I could understand both the audiologist's and my daughter's words right away. From what I've read on the Cochlear Facebook pages, the activation results not only vary from person to person but, as with me, from one implant to another.

I was fortunate to have an iPhone and, following both implants and subsequent activations, it was my primary way to access programs and apps. I learned to interpret the words and sounds from sound waves to something I could identify. I worked at it—2 to 3 hours a day in the beginning. For my first implant, I left my hearing aid out and for the second implant I took off the first processor. Otherwise the brain would go to what it knew instead of being forced into learning this new language. I subscribed to free (through the library) on-line books, and I'd listen while I read the hard copy.

I completed lessons on the phone, via apps, where people talked to me—and then I would answer questions based on what I heard. As I advanced through this process, the sentences changed to paragraphs and then to longer stories... and when that got easy, I would turn off the visual of their faces to avoid reading their lips.

MUSIC: By using a music rehab app called "Bring Back the Beat" I could re-learn one instrument at a time and then begin putting them together. Now with two implants, I not only enjoy music, but I enjoy listening to it in stereo!

In addition to a list of resources for the auditory training process in the back of this book, there's a special music one I highly recommend. If you go to Richard Pocker's Cochlear Implant Basics Home Page. **(link below)** and click on the **"Music Rehab"** tab, you'll find the recordings of many different instruments. I still use this page and enjoy listening to each instrument separately. I know it's helping with my ability to enjoy music again.

https://cochlearimplantbasics.com

Currently I enjoy the music on Richard's website, and I also listen to songs of my choice. If it's a song I'm familiar with, I can usually understand the lyrics…if not, and there are a lot of instruments, it's still difficult. If I'm near my phone or laptop, I look up the lyrics. It's a continuous learning process.

CHAPTER SIX
Sounds
"I didn't know butterfly wings made a sound"

☙

Journal Entry, February 21, 2019
Following February 18 Activation

Whisper...I heard myself whisper this morning!!! Have I ever heard this sound before? Most likely, as otherwise how would I know it was a whisper? I also heard a LOT of background noise in a quiet house...I wonder what that was...I wonder a lot! I'm confident that Dr. Darcy Jaarsma (Grand Rapids audiologist) will be able to adjust the sounds on the 27th...and I'm counting on hearing a whisper without the loud background noise! I still do not understand words unless I am talking out loud to myself...or reading along with an audio book...or the person talking to me tells me (when my hearing aid is on in the right ear) what they are going to be saying...then I turn off my aid & can understand the robotic words via the cochlear on my left side...progress is being made...small steps at a time! Yesterday a friend sang two very familiar songs to me over the telephone...and because I knew the words, and had heard him sing them countless times, I understood them...however, he sounded like Jeremiah (the robotic bullfrog)!

NOTE: I discovered the "loud background noise" was my breathing! Once I knew that, and my brain acknowledged what the sound was, it began to fade. I'm no longer aware of hearing my breathing as background noise

Spring Frogs (Peepers)
Pre-Cochlear Implants, but with Hearing Aids

The songs of spring frogs (peepers) have become one of my favorite sounds. As I wrote in Chapter One, I grew up around water and never heard this sound until after I had Phonak Hearing aids with a wireless Bluetooth microphone. A friend took the microphone down to a swampy area. The sound of peepers was amazing.

About the same time, I was walking in the woods with another friend near some wetlands. This time I heard a sound but could not identify it. I asked my friend—"peepers" was the answer. There was no microphone involved, so the sound was coming directly into my aids. A very different, yet similar, sound from the first time.

And then there was the time a friend and I were canoeing near a lily pond.... I didn't have my wireless microphone but the frogs were loud enough.. They continued singing as we inched the canoe closer. They put on a "leapfrog" show for us that I'll never forget. Not the sound, nor the antics. One little frog

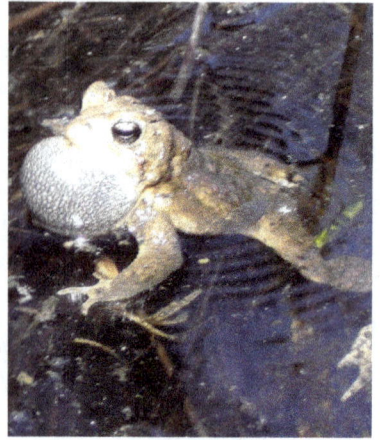

came right over to the side of our canoe, and we were able to see his throat puff up.... All the other frogs were silent as he got ready—then all the frogs joined in the very loud song. Simply amazing!

Hearing Decreased: No More Peeper Sounds

However, my hearing continued to decrease and even with hearing aids and a microphone, the sound of peepers became a thing of the past.

Surprise Return of Peepers' Sounds

Imagine my surprise, when on May 25, 2021, two months after my second implant I once again heard the beloved sound of peepers, I wrote this journal entry:

> *I'm inside...it's cool out, so windows are closed...& I'm HEARING peepers...and what's interesting is that a couple nights ago I heard "sounds" and was trying to figure out what they were. It was only after opening the window that I "got it." Yep, they were peepers...robotic sounding peepers...tonight I sit here and "know" the sounds are coming from the frogs! And they don't sound the least bit robotic!*

Peepers, Wood Frogs, And Chorus Frogs

In writing this, my curiosity got the best of me and I spent some time looking up peepers. I'm not going to put all I learned here, but the most important thing is that there are many different kinds of peepers, with different sounds. That, along with the sound coming directly in the hearing aid versus the microphone, explains why I did not recognize the peeper sound in different environments.

9/28/19 Journal Entry: Baby Chicks

I was blessed to have walked into the Grand Marais Fisheries Farm & Mercantile just as a baby chicken was hatching. What an awesome experience and the timing felt perfect...as this tiny wet creature worked to peck off its shell, and immediately made it's first sounds. I was able to hear both, the shell cracking and the tiny, tiny peeps!

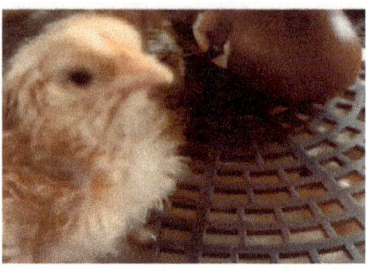

Chicken hatching. Photo courtesy of Brandi Lyn Taylor of Superior Orchards, Grand Marais, Michigan

12-5-21 Journal Entry:

I walked with a friend this morning and laughed with joy when I HEARD the wind rattling the brown leaves of a giant tree....My walking companion identified part of the new sound I was hearing (via my two cochlear implant processors) was the icy snow blowing against the leaves! Amazing!

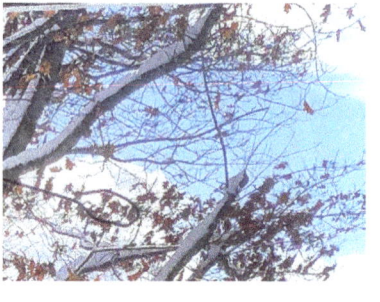

2-6-23 Sounds of Silence as I Write

I've been handwriting my journal entries. Today I decided to write deaf, and I'm observing the total silence. My cat, Boris, is sleeping on my lap.

  I can feel his purr but there is no sound. My pen and hand are moving across the paper but , again, there is no sound. I often

Chapter 7: Sounds

leave my processors off for an hour or two in the morning to just be in the silence, but I've not written with them off until today.

Later today I'll write using the laptop and I plan on taking both processors off to again observe the silence. There will be no keyboard clicking and no printer clacking. What else am I not hearing with the processors removed. My furnace is hot water heat, so I don't hear noise of forced air, but with processors on I do hear the pipes clanging. Not really clanging like the old radiators but dinging as they heat up. Right now, there is no dinging. There is no sound. I can't hear my phone ring. I just took a drink of coffee I did not hear myself sip or slurp, whichever I do. I put the mug down on the ceramic coaster. No sound.

This is interesting, writing about the experience of silence. Side Note: Boris is looking at me and my notebook. I wonder how 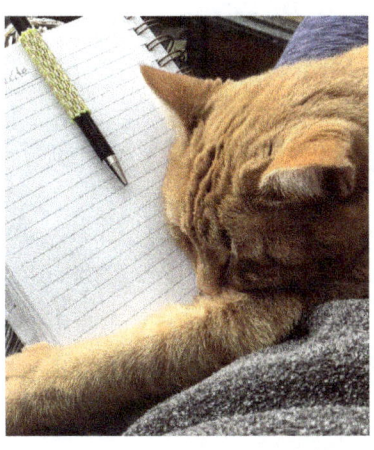 *many writers write with their cat on their lap. The pages flew this morning and I have enjoyed observing silence as I wrote.*

I just put both processors on and, oh my, Boris's purr is so loud after total silence and so very magical, as is the sound of my pen sliding across the paper and my hand moving across it too. Awesome sounds. Now I'm going to take a drink of coffee. I can hear myself sip and I can hear myself swallow. The mug made a delightful sound as I sat it back on the ceramic coaster. I just now heard the hot water heat pipes clicking.

I believe today will be a day of taking processors off and putting them back on and observing. Maybe I'll even snowshoe a bit without them on.

NOTE: I did just that. I snowshoed in the woods without my processors on. While it was interesting to snowshoe and not hear anything…not the click of my poles, the sound of the snow as I stepped, wind in the trees…nothing. I only did this soundless experiment for a couple minutes as, while I'm totally comfortable being deaf in my own house, I did not feel safe in the woods. I wouldn't hear another person coming up behind me, nor an animal. It makes me even more grateful (if that's possible) for the miracle of my implants.

The Sounds of Happy—Cat Purring

The "Sounds of Happy" is what one friend described me hearing my cat purr for the first time. I've had cats for over 20 years and, while I have felt the vibrations of the purr, I heard it for the first time on Sunday, March 3, 2019. Boris was on my lap as I was using my iPhone to do some "hearing lessons." I heard an unfamiliar sound…looked around…nothing different…heard it a few more times before I saw it matched Boris' breathing. Tears flowed as I relished the "sound of happy"—the "sound of peace" (as another friend called it) coming from this beautiful creature.

And a few more sounds…

There have been so many new sounds in the past four plus years, and each one excites me. There are three that stand out as I had no clue that these emitted any sound. That is the wing of the butterfly, dragonfly and hummingbird.

Chapter 7: Sounds

I was standing on the porch of my Grand Marais house and was pleasantly surprised to see a butterfly join me. Then I was even more surprised and touched to know the sound I was now hearing was its wings. **I didn't know that butterfly wings made a sound.** Happy tears flowed.

I also did not know that dragonfly wings and hummingbird wings made sounds. I was with my friend, Darlene, when I first heard, and she identified the sound of the dragonfly wings. I was sitting in my friend, Lisa's, yard when the same thing happened with the sound of hummingbird wings. Such precious hearing moments!

And then there's the squeaky breaks:
My grandson, Mike, recently reminded me of an incident when I was first hearing and identifying new sounds following my first surgery and activation. I heard my brakes squeal before they needed to be replaced before it was metal on metal.

JULY 2023 I am constantly in awe. This past spring, I went camping with my family and left my processors on for a while after I climbed into my tent, as I wanted to hear the sounds of nature. The next morning, I described a bird sound I had not previously heard. I found out it was the whippoorwill doing his mating song.

I'm grateful!

CHAPTER SEVEN
From There to Hear

From Here to There?

From There to Here

☙

Adding to the Team
October 19, 2021

  Where is **There**? Where is **Hear**? And where oh where is **Here**?

  HEAR: The hearing aids I've used, replaced now by my two cochlear implants with two connecting processors, allowing me to HEAR! And to not *only* hear, but to understand the spoken word.

  THERE designates some of the physical and emotional places my hard of hearing journey has taken me as well as some of the places I've lived.

  It is the journey of my progressive hearing loss, which led to the decision to pursue the possibility of cochlear implants. The first implant in 2019 destroyed the little residual hearing I had in my that ear. Up until March 25, 2021, without my cochlear processor attached to my head, I was deaf in my left ear, and had a profound hearing loss in the right, on which I wore a Resound Hearing Aid. The term for one implant and one procrssor combined with one hearing aid is "bimodal."

HERE brings us to the present time, August 2023. After two cochlear implants, I'm considered "bilaterally implanted." Without my processors on my head, I'm "bilaterally deaf." I have complete loss of hearing. *.

Totally and completely deaf until I put on one or both cochlear processors and they connect to the implant, magnet to magnet, taking sounds to the receiver inside my head. and thereby to the electrode array, which circles around the cochlea. My brain translates these electrical impulses into understandable spoken words.

The more I work on my audio rehab/auditory training "brain training exercises" (even four plus years after the first implant) the more I improve on how well I understand not only the spoken word, but the environmental sounds around me as well. Most conversations have become easy, with an occasional new word or phrase that may need to be clarified with the speaker. After repeating this word/phrase a few times, my brain will recognize it. I still need to ask some people to slow down and then, often clarify that slowing down does not mean speaking louder. Sometimes I feel I'm experiencing a bit of congitive delay between when the word is spoken and when it's correctly translated by my brain. I notice this most in group converations.

Chapter 7: From There to Hear & From Hear to There

I do not do well in noise. Part of that is because I live alone and my exposure to noise is minimal; therefore, there's fewer opportunities for brain training. I have programs on my phone to practice listening to words and sentences within noise. However, since I'm not exposed to real-time noise on a regular basis, I believe these artificial background noises have not been of much help—or maybe I've not used them enough.

When I'm in a group setting and several different conversations are going on, I understand very little. I've often asked family and friends to please let me know when plans are being made that I need to be aware of—otherwise I've found that people are getting on coats to head out somewhere and I have no clue where we are going. It's important for the hard of hearing person to advocate for themselves, ensuring others know their needs. it's also important to have patience, as others simply need reminders of our invisible disability. If we had a cast or brace on, or were using crutches or a wheelchair, they would have a visible reminder we may need help.

*NOTE: *I want to add a side note here for anyone contemplating a cochlear implant. While many cochlear surgeries do leave the patient completely deaf in the implanted ear(s), some people do retain a degree of residual hearing and can wear a hybrid processor, which combines the sound from the implant and the residual sound. My surgeon had warned me this would not be happening in my case.*

Living In a Rural Remote Area

I had been traveling the 700-mile round trip to Grand Rapids, MI from Grand Marais, MI for about five years for pre-cochlear implant evaluations and other necessary appointments, the two surgeries, and very frequent post-op appointments with the surgeon and audiologist. With my move to Upper Michigan's Keweenaw Peninsula, in the summer of 2021, the distance has increased, to a round trip over 1,000 miles.

New Audiology Opportunity

Until recently, all of Michigan's Upper Peninsula (UP) cochlear implant candidates needed to travel to somewhere out of the UP for evaluations, surgery, and the very important "mappings." There were not (*and, as of this writing, still are not*) any surgeons in the UP who could perform the operation. And, until recently, there were no UP audiologists trained in doing the testing, the important activation, nor the frequent mapping for the implants.

This has changed with Upper Peninsula Audiology, based in Iron Mountain and Houghton, now offering cochlear implant services. I found out about this new service and about their cochlear specialist, Dr. Kati Stilwell, and was excited to know there might be a possibility of less travel time for adjustments.

However, I was apprehensive. I've worked exclusively with Dr. Darcy Jaarsma, AuD, CCC-A, of Spectrum Hospital's Audiology department from the first testing in 2018 to the most recent "mapping." She was the one who "turned on the sound" four plus years ago after the first implant. When I watch the video my daughter took of that momentous day, I still cry. Was

I ready to trade in the years of Dr. Darcy's awesome, skilled service for a new audiologist?

Exploring all options by talking with my surgeon, Dr. Daniels, as well as with Dr. Darcy and Dr. Kati, we decided I didn't need to give anything up, but just add Dr. Kati to the team. I want to tell you that both Dr. Darcy and Dr. Kati were very excited to do this, and both were present at my October 19, 2021, mapping, which took place at Spectrum Hospital in Grand Rapids. Dr. Kati attended remotely from Houghton and not only could we see her, but she and Dr. Darcy shared computer screens. Dr. Kati could see every electronic adjustment Dr. Darcy made.

I am so excited to know that if I should have an issue with the implant/processors in-between appointments with Dr. Darcy, I can call Dr. Kati and schedule an appointment 30 minutes from my house. Dr. Darcy will share her files with Dr. Kati and can attend remotely.

Dr Marlene Bevan, founder/director of Audiocare Hearing Centers in Traverse City and Gaylord, Michigan shared with me that there are more audiologists joining the network of folks involved in delivering quality services to cochlear recipients now than when I initially sought help.

Cochlear America has developed a Cochlear Provider Network, of which Dr. Bevan is a member, both to educate and support clinical audiologists. Now more than ever help is available.

Things just keep getting better.

CHAPTER EIGHT
And then there's the rough spots…

☙

With any surgery there's always a chance of some not-fun after effects. And with any implanted device, whether it's heart, kidney, knee…, or a cochlear implant, there's always the chance of some negative side effects. And, while it's rare, there's also the chance the body will reject the implanted item.

I'm going to write about a few of my interesting aftereffects, all of which have either dissipated, or no longer bother me. I only include this because I had some unexpected challenges, even with all the research I did prior to both of my surgeries. I simply want to bring a level of awareness to some possible issues and solutions, and hopefully help diminish fears of the unknown.

The Wayward Electrode

Following my first activation in 2019, I experienced some shooting pain in my head on the implanted side. This pain was more intense with certain sounds, one that sounded like the ravens who lived in the woods next to my house. I reported this to my audiologist and at my next appointment, I was able to pinpoint the sound as she tested each electrode. Once we identified the sound, Dr. Darcy Jaarsma, began turning down that particular electrode, however with no positive effect on the electrical jolt I was experiencing. Dr. Darcy disconnected the errant electrode, with no adverse consequences to my hearing ability.

I was also experiencing brain fog, and with the disconnection of the electrode this, the headaches and sudden jolts dissipated. Upon returning home, the ravens still sounded like ravens, now without the pain I had been experiencing.

Grief, *Only a Few Instances*

While I have had some intermittent sadness associated with my hearing loss, I have only experienced intense grief a couple times.

Once when I needed to turn down a coveted reporting job, and then when I realized and accepted my hearing loss had progressed to the point where even the best hearing aids on the market were not enough. And when I discovered "total deafness" meant I could not hear my own voice!

As mentioned in a previous chapter, while I thought I was prepared to be deaf following my second implant, I had no idea what that really meant! Therefore, it was a harsh moment when, following the second surgery, as my daughter was changing the battery on the processor of my previously implanted side, (which I couldn't reach as it was taped to my bandage) I began to talk to her and was in absolute shock to realize deaf meant I could not hear my own voice.

All the above instances of grief were harsh, but short-lived. With the realization of what deaf meant, I slipped into incredible sadness. This was alleviated with a call from my

Chapter 8: And then there's the rough spots...

daughter, Beth, to her brother, Tom. Tom is noted for his hilarious made-up songs. She told him, "Mom's having a really rough time, can you sing to her?" And he did. He and my daughter-in-law/friend, Sue, were out at their camp. He grabbed an ax for a pretend microphone and Sue videoed him singing his very own rendition of "A Sound of Silence." What could I do when I saw that? Laugh, that's what! And watch it over and over and laugh and laugh. The very best medicine.

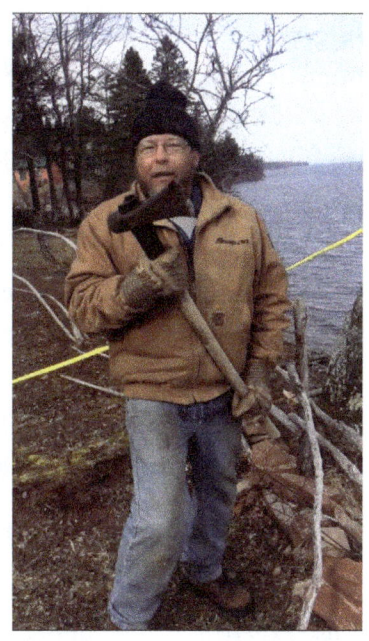

Later I began experimenting with the total silence. I'd leave my processors off for periods of time. I'd watch my cat meow for food, with his mouth wide open but no sound coming out. I'd giggle every time!

I continue to experiment with my world of silence. I am still in awe that, with the simple act of putting on my processors, I can hear. They come off, I'm completely deaf. What a wonderful invention the cochlear implant is!

Vertigo

Following my first implant, I had some major attacks of vertigo, making me dizzy and nauseated, sometimes unable to get out of bed for days. The vertigo was an aftereffect of surgery, which caused small crystals of calcium to come loose in my inner ear.

My surgeon gave me a sheet of paper with guidelines for the Epley Maneuver. However, I could not do these as they made me dizzier and more nauseated.

NOTE: I've read on the Cochlear Facebook groups where many cochlear implant recipients have had great success with the Epley Maneuver, as certain actions can move the calcium crystals out of your semi-circular canal, often bringing relief.

For whatever reason, vertigo is no longer an issue. I guess the calcium crystals took care of themselves.

A Bit Off Balance

I also experienced a bit of loss of balance. As luck would have it my daughter's friend, Jacque taught a program called "Brains in Motion." She stopped over and learning of my balance issues, invited me to her class, which focused on balance. She worked with me and gifted me with a bag of bouncing balls and lessons as to how to use them. While I know using them helped my balance issues, some lingering issues, which might be caused by the surgeries—or maybe just my age, remain. Writing this is a good reminder for me to get the balls out of the bag, rewatch the videos and do the exercises.

While Jacque no longer teaches this class, she has referred me to a website

https://www.bal-a-vis-x.com

Bal-A-Vis-X is an acronym for Balance/Auditory/ Vision eXercises, all of which are deeply rooted in rhythm.

Chapter 8: And then there's the rough spots...

Tinnitus

Tinnitus is a variety of sound that is heard when no corresponding external sound is present. Wikipedia:

According to studies at Mayo Clinic cochlear implants have reduced and/or increased tinnitus.

https://www.mayoclinic.org/tests-procedures/ cochlear-implants/about/pac-20385021

I'm going to address some tinnitus related aftereffects, which I experienced. Some of which I didn't tell anyone about until I had read on the Cochlear Facebook sites that others had the same experiences. I certainly didn't want anyone to think I was crazy.

I've personally experienced three different kinds of tinnitus since receiving my implants. While two still exist, they do not cause me any distress.

Pulsatile Tinnitus

The first one I experienced was shortly after my first surgery. I heard drumming. Steady drumming. I was living in Grand Marais, MI, on the ridge above town. I knew a friend had recently been drumming at a park on the point of the harbor. So, when I first heard this "drumming," I figured it was him and most likely others, as the sound was traveling a good distance. Then, when it continued into the evening, I was concerned that some townspeople would be concerned over the "noise." I called my friend on his cell phone. He was home. He had not been drumming. So, I paid more attention to the drumming, which

I was still hearing. It matched my heartbeat. I immediately did some online research and discovered that it was most likely Pulsatile Tinnitus, which I figured had nothing to do with any major vein malfunction, but rather the swelling that was still present from my surgery. As the swelling receded the "heartbeat drumming sound" dissipated, never to return.

Again, I have read on the Cochlear Facebook pages, where others have also experienced this interesting side effect.

NOTE: if you are experiencing this type of tinnitus out of the blue, or if it persists, please seek medical help.

Roaring Tinnitus

This is a rather common form of tinnitus, and one I still experience occasionally since getting implanted. The roaring is never a loud enough roar to cause distress, and it always disappears as soon as I put on my processors. It usually occurs first thing in the morning before I put on my processors.

Musical Ear Syndrome or maybe
Newscasting Tinnitus:

While I've not found "Newscasting Tinnitus" listed in my online searches, I have found Musical Ear Syndrome, which seems to have the same characteristics.

I told no one about this experience for a long time… hearing a far-off news radio broadcast? Voices not recognizable, but there? And then I became aware of people on the Cochlear Facebook

Chapter 8: And then there's the rough spots...

pages, posting their experiences with this phenomenon. Ah, I was not crazy!

As with the other two tinnitus experiences, I only experience it when both processors are off and it is so far in the distance that it causes me no stress. The "newscast" disappears as soon as I put on one or both processors. From what I've read, something like the phantom feelings amputees sometimes get following the removal of a limb, these sounds could be the brain trying to hear, relying on past sound memory.

Fast Forward to August, 2023

It's more than five years since I began my journey into exploring the possibilities of getting cochlear implants. Four plus years since my first implant and over two years since my second. Any and all of the side effects are so minimal to me compared with the ability to hear and understand the spoken word. Presently I'm experiencing the magical sounds of summer in Michigan's Upper Peninsula.

CHAPTER NINE
Other Perspectives

January 10, 2020:
From Daughter Beth:

It's been one year since my number one **GRITT** girl had her cochlear implant. 366 days ago her hearing was at 34% recognition with the highest powered top of the line hearing aids, 0% without. She had the **Guts** at 76 to take the challenge, **Resilience** to recover from major surgery to the head, her **Invincible** spirit kept her studying and practicing to retrain her brain to translate the robotic sounds into words, being a **Team** player she's writing a book to tell her story in hopes to convince others to prepare and take the journey, and the **Tenacity** not to give up and has worked so hard that she now has 95% recognition of spoken words! <u>**Carol Rose**</u>, you are a true GRITT girl! I'm the lucky girl who gets to call you mom. I love you and am so proud of who you are and what you continue to help me become!!!

FROM THERE TO HEAR

Grandma's Hearing Loss & Cochlear Implants
by Stephanie Tavill

When I think of my grandma I think of her involvement with the non-profit, Keweenaw Krayons, at which I spent a good part of my childhood. I also remember time spent visiting playgrounds, gardening, testing chicken strips at every local restaurant, and unconditional love. I think about the strong friendship and love we share as adults. I don't think about hearing loss, though to say it didn't influence many of our interactions would be a lie.

When she moved to the Keweenaw, I was still quite young. Her house had a hidden storage area under the eaves, and it was the perfect size for kids to play. I was in a big Harriet the Spy phase, and she had an old typewriter up in the storage area. I would pretend to be a writer, like I knew my grandma had been back in Traverse City, and "type" up my spy stories hidden away in that secret room.

I also clearly remember the special gizmos and gadgets she had in that home to support her as a hearing-impaired person living alone. She had lights, which would blink on and off if someone rang the doorbell or called her phone. She had Mandy, a dog who had the intentions of being a hearing dog, but instead was just a great friend. When we had sleepovers, we would have to wake grandma up in the mornings by tapping her or turning the light on and off. Without her hearing aids in, she wouldn't know that my brothers and I were up and wreaking havoc on her house.

My favorite "gadget" was her microphone. When she got the microphone, I felt like her hearing really improved. My brothers and I would take turns hanging the microphone around our necks and talking into it while out and about on our various adventures. We still had to repeat ourselves a lot, but the microphone made things better. I recall one particular meal at a restaurant where my brothers and I were having a conversation, which was not meant for Grandma's ears. She had stepped away to use the restroom but had left her microphone on the table. When we saw the microphone on the table mid-conversation, we were mortified that she had been listening in. But when she came back to the table, we realized that she hadn't heard it at all. Even with her microphone she struggled when we were in places with a lot of background noise. Other times when we would be out with Grandma, and she stepped away to use the restroom we would grab her microphone and put it close to our mouths and make farting noises. Of course, we failed to remember that only grandma could hear the noises and not the entire restroom. But we still thought we were pretty funny.

We learned to talk a bit slower, be patient, and repeat ourselves as needed. It wasn't really until I was an adult that her hearing started to have a more profound impact on our social interactions. It was obvious that she wasn't following the story as the family sat around talking at a fire pit or playing games. I was very excited when she shared with us that she was going to get cochlear implants. I knew it would bring her back into the conversation, something we all wanted. I was excited and I knew she was too, but she couldn't hide the fact that she was also scared about the whole process. My grandma is an incredibly brave and strong woman, who climbs ice cliffs, canoes, and hikes now into her 80s. I knew that it was taking her a great deal of that bravery to undergo this surgery.

FROM THERE TO HEAR

Since Grandma got the cochlear implants, our conversations are definitely improved. During a visit to Florida, we were riding bikes on the beach. There was wind, waves, and the sounds of families enjoying themselves. While we biked my grandma and I were able to talk to one another. I was blown away by the fact that she could understand me despite all of the background noise and without reading my lips. Since her cochlear implants, we talk much more on the phone, and she gets to enjoy watching her great-grandchildren grow through Facetime. She can even understand the playful talk of a two-year-old who doesn't always get the words quite right. I'm grateful for the enrichment that my grandma's cochlear implants have brought to her life and our family.

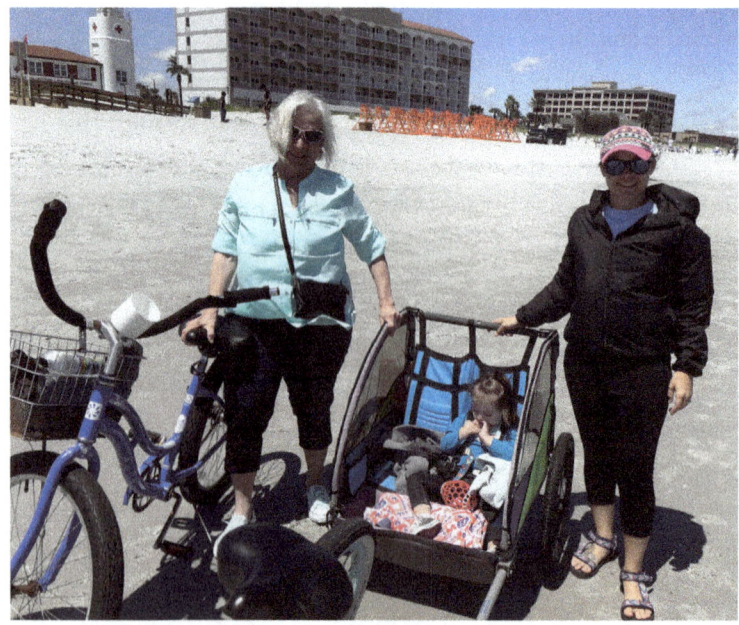

Chapter 9: Other Perspectives

From Friend Darlene:

When I had to practice how I spoke to be an on-air radio news person for Minnesota Public Radio's station in Houghton, I never knew it was good training for how to be a friend to two very special people in my life who had progressive hearing loss.

I met Carol Rose while she still had hearing aids, and learned, with her help, to be sure to face her while I was talking with her, and to speak clearly, with pauses to help with understanding. My voice timbre helped, as it matched with the best hearing one for both friends.

As the years went on, and the hearing loss increased, we navigated the best ways to keep communication clear and as easy as possible. The advantage I had as a friend was that Carol Rose was very good at expressing what she needed me to do to help that along. My part was to be conscious of her hearing needs and follow them as best as humanly possible. We both struggled at times but had laughter to help us out of the most challenging situations.

What I did not realize was how severely her hearing loss had become before she decided to get the first cochlear implant. I felt she was not wanting others to know, or perhaps even herself, how much hearing loss was affecting every aspect of her life. At that time I was living a 4-hour drive away and we spent time on the phone, with occasional visits. If I'm remembering correctly, the phone visits were easier, but I'm not exactly sure why that was so.

Her courage to go ahead, with especially the first cochlear implant, was astounding! She was living alone, in a rural setting with harsh winters, and had to have someone come and snow blow her driveway so she could get out to drive 8 hours downstate.

While her family was a huge support during the whole process, she needed to re-learn how to hear/listen with the implant once she was back "on the Ridge." Our phone calls were part of the practice, until she needed real connection and would put the hearing aid back in her other ear for that part. My part was to understand as best I could what she was going through and be part of her re-learning process as a friend on the phone. And offer whatever encouragement and support I could from afar.

This woman I call friend is an amazing human being, and an all-around advocate for herself and others with profound hearing loss. She took on the technology—even before the implants—as it became available to her, and she found ways to work with the system to be sure she received the help she needed to keep going as a reporter for the local newspaper in the town she was in—until she could not.

That's when, along with her visit to the audiologist, she began to realize that her options were narrowing. Hearing aids didn't work for her anymore. Cochlear implants were what would give her back her life—a quality life with family and friends and community. At that point, she bravely made the decision to go ahead with the cochlear implant, and she continues to this day to camp and garden and hear her great grands as part of her growing family and laugh and share writing and be open to life at its hearing best for her and those around her!

I feel privileged to keep learning along with her, and to call her my friend, and I am so glad she keeps choosing the best hearing options no matter how hard or challenging, to allow all of us the reward of her.

Darlene, a friend for the past 25 years

Chapter 9: Other Perspectives

Thoughts from a friend of 23 years
By Len Novak

I've learned from Carol of the meaningfulness of patience in communicating with a hard of hearing person. I have certainly come to know, through Carol's assertive ways, that when asking someone to repeat something she means she really wants to hear it, whatever it is, and saying "never mind" can crush the spirit of a hard of hearing person.

Getting the hard of hearing person to understand may take multiple repetitions, and possibly rewording the statement.

Spunk is something I love, respect and appreciate in a friend and I can tell you that Carol's level of spunk capability in getting people to understand the needs of a hard of hearing person has evolved incredibly. I also understand the energy it takes to keep being proactive.

I hope the many hard of hearing readers of this book will have the opportunity to find a friend, if they don't have one, who is willing to find the patience (at least sometimes) and has the capacity to encourage, solicit and respect the spunk it can take to ask for help.

I often get excited when I speak and talk too loud and too fast for Carol. She has no trouble interrupting me to ask me to speak quieter and slower. I must say that after 19 years of knowing her when she wore hearing aids and I needed to speak up, till the past four years of having cochlear implants, where I need to keep my voice lowered, has been a learning experience for me.

Carol and I have a lifetime commitment to friendship and during this lifetime I will continue to remind myself to be aware of the level and speed of my voice as I communicate.

FROM THERE TO HEAR

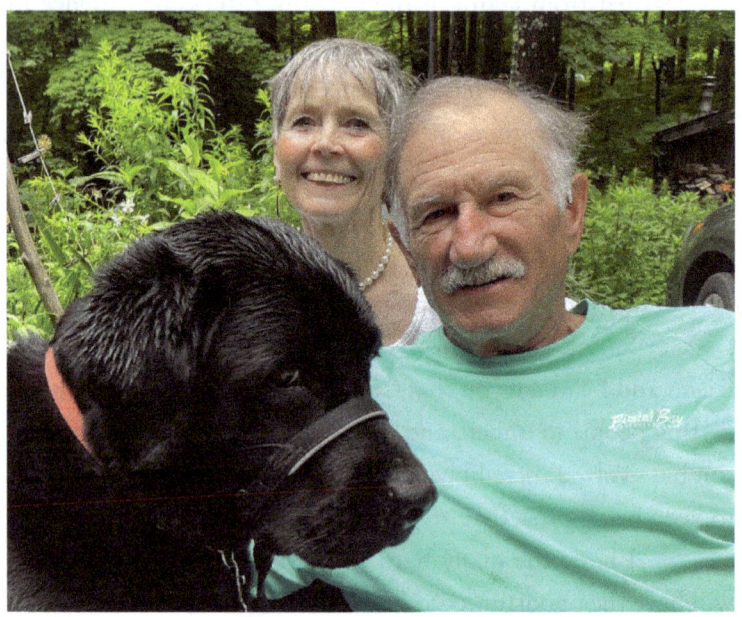

Note from Carol Rose: *I thank Margaret Gerhard for sharing about Team Andy, and I hope her story will help you decide if a hearing dog is meant to be in your life. Can Do Canines currently only operate in Wisconsin and Minnesota. I've put their webpage info at the end of this chapter and also the webpages of other hearing dog resources.*

CHAPTER TEN
Is a Hearing Assist Dog Right for You?

҉

Hearing Assist Dogs (HAD)
Team Andy by Margaret Gerhard

We are honored and proud to introduce you to "TEAM ANDY"

"Team Andy" involves three members: Andy, Steve and me, Margaret, Steve's wife of 45 years.

Andy, our certified HAD trained service dog is devoted to his master Steve, a Vietnam veteran and bilateral cochlear implant recipient.

As a young man, Steve served our country spraying agent orange and dropping bombs from helicopters for 14 months as part of an army chemical detachment. In addition to unresolved, perplexing painful and unusual skin eruptions, Steve lost his hearing.

After years of struggling, a young health clinic audiologist working as an intern, suggested he might be an eligible candidate for cochlear implant surgery. It couldn't be any worse than what he experienced in the war, right? He decided to go for it! He had his first cochlear surgery in the spring of 2011. About

18 months later his second surgery was scheduled. Both surgeries went well. He experienced minimal dizziness and nausea, no vertigo and managed his pain with the prescribed medications.

Following the implants, Steve worked training his brain to hear differently by watching tv and talking to himself, talking to the loons, the fish, the lake, the trees and the big blue sky when he went fishing in the early morning hours on our little lake.

Part of having cochlear implants and the accompanying devices is tending to the necessary care and maintenance of these miraculous external assists. The processors need to be cleaned and the batteries charged regularly. Typically, that is a nightly requirement. While some people with cochlear implants retain a degree of residual hearing, many are totally deaf in the implanted ear.

Steve did not retain any residual hearing and therefore, after his second implant, he was totally deaf. Without his processors on, he hears nothing. When the processors, which are connected via a magnet to the implant, are off his head, while cleaning them or sleeping, he hears nothing!

He cannot hear a late-night phone call, the doorbell or knock at the door, fire, smoke or carbon monoxide alarms, someone yelling an alert, or an intruder etc. It's a very vulnerable position to be in!

This is not as much of an issue if the user has an attentive (light sleeper!) hearing soul constantly in the household to alert them to these sounds and potentially dangerous situations. In our case Steve is alone when I am on the road traveling, frequently overnight. It was a constant worry for me to leave him. I prayed he would be safe.

Chapter 10: Is a Hearing Assist Dog Right for You?

All that changed with the arrival of our WONDER, as in WONDERFUL, service dog Andy! Andy is a handsome 63 pound HAD trained black lab! He is a recent graduate of Can Do Canines in New Hope, Minnesota.

Learning about this organization in New Hope certainly gave us NEW HOPE! (Aptly named location for this nonprofit organization!) We promptly filled out the paperwork, submitted a single $50 application fee, and waited. Within a short time, we had a phone interview with a Client Services Coordinator. Since this was during Covid, we had several introductory, informative zoom meetings, and then zoom training sessions.

Finally, just days before Christmas in 2021, we received a call that Can Do Canines had a possible match for Steve! A dog named Andy was available! What a Christmas gift this news was for us!

Even more affirming for us was when we received a call in January asking if we could come meet Andy! This was just days before Steve's late January birthday! We saw this as another positive sign from the universe! The stars were aligned! Prayers were being answered! We drove to Minnesota to meet Andy! It was love at first sight!

So there in NEW HOPE at the end of January we had several days of thorough on-site campus and community training. We went with Andy and our Client Services Coordinator to area restaurants and shopping malls to practice entering elevators, etc.

We learned how the team was to work together in public situations.

We spent the nights in our motel, bonding with Andy! We were then sent home with Andy and a generous tote bag of goodies, gear, toys, food, and a client manual. The client manual is a very helpful, detailed resource instruction handbook. It includes the hotline and personal home texting number for our specific Can Do Canine Client Services Coordinator in case we have any immediate, urgent concerns! (Now that is dedication!)

Andy had an easy time acclimating to our home and surroundings, He came to us potty trained, knew 33 different commands and adjusted well living with his new roommate, a chubby male cat named Gray the Stray!

Our Client Services Coordinator made several home visits, did additional training, gave tips and took video recordings to evaluate Team Andy's progress and training in his new home environment.

Finally, Team Andy passed the required tests. The team attended Andy's graduation in New Hope at the campus!

Andy adds a greater sense of security in our loves, a deeper peace of mind. He is such a blessing. He is a joy. Andy's antics and expressions humor us! He eases stress in the home, great for PTSD relief. Steve and Andy are special buddies to each other.

Recently Steve received a brand-new ankle, a surgery, which resulted in 12 weeks of constant bed rest and rehab therapy. Andy was a true healer and constant bedside companion, a welcome pain diversion, easing stress during Steve's recovery.

During this time Andy not only alerted Steve by a nudge on the thigh when the phone, alarms and doorbell rang, he also retrieved Steve's cane, sock or book when it fell and gave it back to him.

Andy played messenger, taking written notes to and

from me when I was in other parts of the house, where Steve could not hear me from his hospital bed. Andy diligently delivered these notes.

WE ARE SO GRATEFUL TO THE DEDICATED STAFF AT CAN DO CANINES!

We share our Can Do Canines' story here in the hopes it will encourage other cochlear implant users to consider an assistive service dog to keep you and your loved ones safe when "unplugged" from your cochlear implant.

Be assured Can Do Canines will match you and your dog according to YOUR needs, your personality, your lifestyle and yes, even your size!

It might be a relief to know that not everyone gets a 63-pound black lab bundle of love! Smaller dogs are available!

Please spread the word that Can Do Canines not only serves clients with hearing loss, but others with mobility issues, autism, seizure disorders, and Type I diabetes.

Steve and I highly recommend Can Do Canines which serves clients in Wisconsin and Minnesota. There are other fine organizations as well, many which can be found on the resources list below:

Assistance dogs can give the people who need them more freedom, independence, and peace of mind while living that life.

Happy Trails, Happy Tails
Resources:
candocanines.org
assistancedogsinternational.org
https://www.pawswithacause.org

FROM THERE TO HEAR

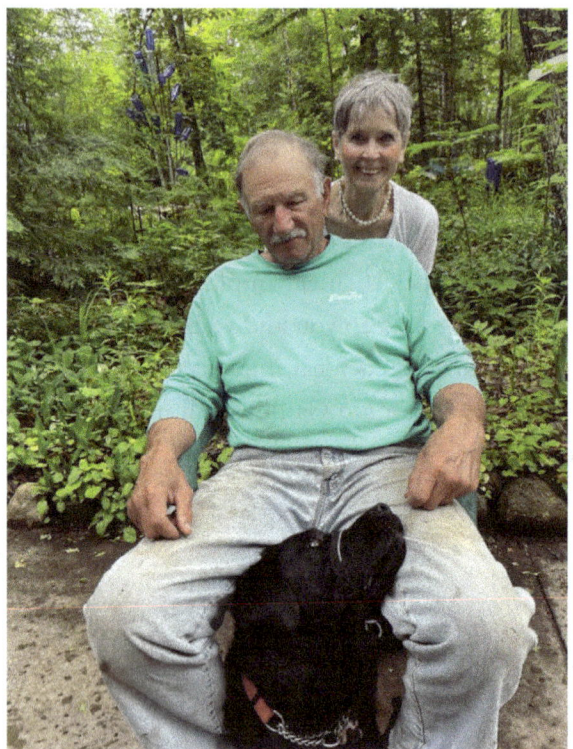

One of Andy's favorite commands, which he loves to do is "PARK." This command means he very swiftly and adeptly backs up and scoots under the chair where Steve is sitting. Andy is tucked under the chair and safely out of pedestrian's way.

NOTE from Carol Rose : If you are hard of hearing or deaf, please contact your local fire department or the Red Cross as there may be help available for smoke alarms with loud volume, flashing lights and/or bed shakers. I was a recent grateful recipient of such a system from Red Cross.

Acknowledgements

A huge shout out to the medical staff who have been there for me over the years. Because they are all equally important, and my life would not be the same without any one of them, I'm listing them in alphabetical order according to their last names. *Carol Rose*

Marlene A. Bevan, Ph.D
Audiologist
Founder/Director Audicare Hearing Centers
Traverse City and Gaylord, MI
Provides cochlear candidacy evaluations and follow-up care to cochlear implant recipients in Northern Michigan.

Melissa Collard Au.D., CCC-A
Owner & Audiologist at Upper Peninsula Audiology, Inc.
Houghton and Iron Mountain, Michigan

Robert Daniels, MD
and Staff, especially his nurse, Carol
ENT Center
Grand Rapids and Byron Center, MI

Jackie Gilbert, MS, CCC-A
Audiologist
Superior Ear, Nose & Throat Specialist
Marquette, Michigan

FROM THERE TO HEAR

Valeta Gage
    Graduate of the School of Clinical Sciences
    Speech, Language, and Hearing Sciences Program
    Northern Michigan University
    Currently a Central Michigan University Speech
    Language Pathology Master's Student

Heather Isaacson, Ed.S., CCC-SLP
    Assistant Professor
    School of Clinical Sciences
    Speech, Language, and Hearing Sciences Program
    Northern Michigan University

Darcy Jaarsma, AuD, CCC-A
    Audiologist
    Corewell Health, Grand Rapids, MI
    Note: *Corewell Health was Spectrum Health when I began working with Darcy in 2018*

Brian Kuopus, Audiologist
    Superior Hearing, Marquette, MI

Nancy Reed, Retired Audiologist
    Hancock, Michigan

Kati Stilwell, Au.D., CCC-A
    Audiologist, Specializing in Cochlear Implants
    Upper Peninsula Audiology
    Houghton & Iron Mountain, MI

Acknowledgements

Outreach

I firmly believe it is our responsibility as deaf/hard of hearing people to continue to educate the world at large, as they are open to being educated, about our invisible disability. This is why I enjoyed my previous role as Hearing Technology Resources Specialist (HTRS), a volunteer position with the Michigan Chapter of Hearing Loss Association of America. We demoed assistive technology for the hard of hearing. The awesome program came to an end due to lack of continued funding. I missed it.

Therefore, I was beyond excited when, several years ago, my audiologist, Jackie Gilbert, referred me to Heather Isaacson, Assistant Professor of the School of Clinical Sciences Speech, Language, and Hearing Sciences Program at Northern Michigan University, who asked if I would be interested in speaking to her class.

I was thrilled and I did the first couple presentations in person. The students were interested, and I believe enjoyed learning from a hard of hearing person. Then Covid hit and we began doing the presentations via Zoom. Heather was a skilled host, and the classes ran smoothly. I was able to interact with each student as if I were in the room. Valeta Gage was a student in one of those classes and she decided she wanted more exploration of the rehabilitation and auditory development after a cochlear implant surgery. She contacted me and we set up Zoom meetings, where she would work with me on auditory rehab projects, which she created.

"I was able to learn more about you and your story, which has allowed me to be more gracious with my clients now and able to take a different perspective," she recently wrote.

FROM THERE TO HEAR

"Learning about the technology and process of cochlear implants was so incredibly interesting and it was amazing to learn from the perspective of one going through it."

Val is Currently a Central Michigan University Speech Language Pathology Master's Student.

A SIDE STORY: I was scheduled to speak to the class in early 2023 and I had it marked on my calendar. I even sent a reminder to myself the day before so I would have all my notes ready. I was to sign on to Zoom at 8:45am; 15 minutes early in order to connect with Heather before the students joined us. When my phone rang at 9am and I was it was Heather, it was one of those "oh no" moments! While I had remembered the day before, I had completely forgotten the morning of the class. I asked Heather's forgiveness and said I could join in 10 minutes. That worked for her.

I started my presentation with the story of sliding into class late because I had forgotten. I'm sure some of the students identified with having done this sometime in their college life as I received a lot of knowing smiles.

The class, as usual, was awesome. Extremely interactive with well-thought-out questions for me. After the class I was pleased to receive this note from Heather.

"Hi Carol. My students had to write a reflection of their learning from listening to your story. The summary is... they loved hearing your story and they believe that you are one of the best guest speakers they've heard in all of their time at NMU! "

The reason for this story is not to pat myself on the back, but to urge all of you to reach out, help educate people to

Acknowledgements

the invisible disability of hearing loss. Share about the ways you have made your life better with the use of hearing aids, cochlear implants, Baha implants or other assistive technology. And remember to gently remind them how they can be of help.

More Thank Yous

I could fill this whole book with thank yous as there are so many special people who have assisted me in this journey. If I begin I know I'd leave out someone very important, so please know that whatever it was you did that helped me to hear and understand the spoken word and sounds, it is appreciated more than you'll ever know. Love, Carol Rose.

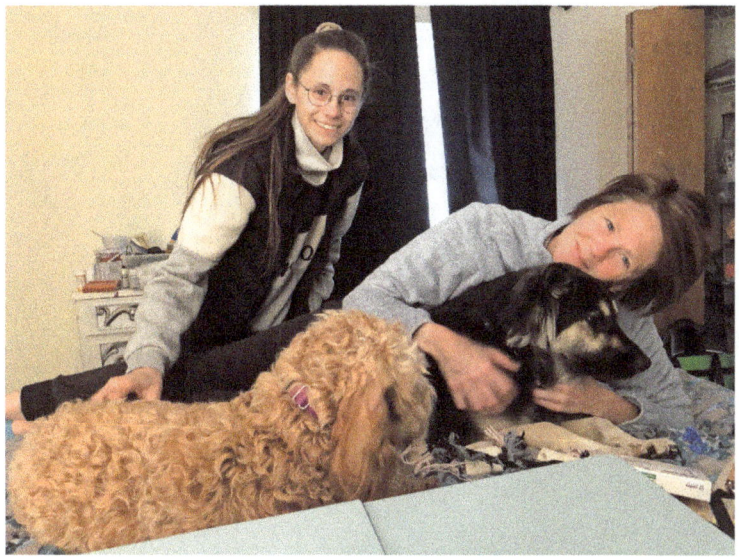

Special thanks to my primary post-surgery and early auditory rehab caregivers, Mena and Beth, along with Stella and Stevie.

Glossary

Here's a few definitions of some of the words in the book, which might be unfamiliar to you. This is in no way meant to be conclusive and I urge you to do your own research.

Americans with Disabilities Act (ADA) of 1990 provides comprehensive civil rights protections to individuals with disabilities in the areas of employment, state and local government services, public accommodations, transportation, and telecommunications.

Electrode Array
An electrode array is the essential part of a cochlear implant (CI). It is inserted into the cochlea of the inner ear in the near proximity of auditory nerve fibers and allows their electrical stimulation.

Epley Maneuver
A series of head movement to relieve symptoms of benign positional vertigo.

Mapping See pages 40 and 41

Nonsyndromic Hearing Loss is a partial or total loss of hearing that is not associated with other signs and symptoms.

Sensorineural Hearing loss (SNHL)
The most common type of permanent hearing, it causes sounds to become unclear or muffled sounding. It may be caused by inner ear damage or problems with the nerve pathways and in some cases, the etiology (cause) may remain unknown.

Additional Resources

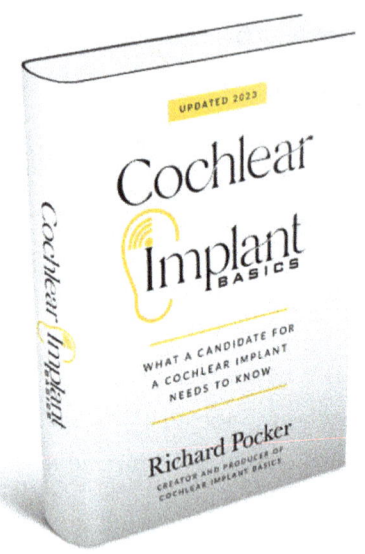

Cochlear Implant Basics:
The Information on the next few pages is taken, with permission of Richard Pocker, from his book and Facebook page, *Cochlear Implant Basics.* Also inside his book is part of his story and interviews with other cochlear implant candidates, recipients, surgeons and other professionals. Thanks, Richard, for your tireless effort in advocating for the deaf and hard of hearing and allowing me to share some of your information here.

Additional Resources from Cochlear Implant Basics by Richard Pocker

Rehabilitation Techniques

Note: Live links are found at cochlearimplantbasics.com

Tips for Cochlear Implant and BAHA Rehabilitation

Your hearing journey begins the day of your activation. Though that first day of restored hearing is filled with much anticipation, emotion, and joy it is important to remember your hearing will most likely not be instantly "normal" nor equivalent to others' hearing experience. Just as no two people are alike, no two journeys into the world of cochlear implant hearing will be alike. What others have found helpful may not work for you. Some of these exercises require a helper (a hearing partner) to read and score your responses. <u>If you don't have a hearing partner on your journey,</u> don't worry. <u>Most of these suggestions can be done alone.</u>

NEVER COMPARE your hearing journey with that of others.

Many Cochlear Implant recipients will tell you that the **three P's—practice, patience, and perseverance-** will determine how well you hear. Please understand that having the mindset of "low expectations and high hopes" will spare you from disappointment and frustration during those early days of hearing.

Repetition, repetition, repetition!!!

Your hearing journey is ongoing your comprehension of speech and sounds will improve significantly over time. Learning to hear with a cochlear implant or BAHA is a skills development exercise like any other: the more you practice and commit to an exceptional hearing outcome, the better your hearing comprehension will improve. At times, this may be emotionally taxing and perhaps even frustrating, but recipients routinely create exceptional hearing outcomes by investing the required time and energy.

DO NOT GET DISCOURAGED. ATTITUDE IS 90% OF THE PATH TO SUCCESS.

This is a compilation of what other CI recipients, and I have found helpful in our hearing journeys.

- **Relax!!!** Your hearing journey is a marathon not a sprint. Just as an athlete conditions for her event you must also condition your brain to interpret the new sounds you're hearing.
- Do not set a timetable as to what and when you're going to understand the different sounds around you. Your listening comprehension will improve on a timeline that is unique to you.
- Let the sounds come to you.
- Look at everyday as a new day filled with **WOW** moments.
- Wear your processor all day. If you feel tired, overwhelmed by sound, or your hearing seems a little off it's fine to "rest "by taking off your processor for a short period of time. Giving your brain short breaks is just as beneficial as giving it a good workout.

Additional Resources from Cochlear Implant Basics by Richard Pocker

- Close your eyes and take yourself to that "peaceful" place far away from the pressure to perfectly understand everything you hear.
- Keep the television or radio on all day. Using the wireless accessories will vastly improve sound. There will be no distortion nor interference from Wi-Fi networks, mobile phones, etc.
- Watch programs and movies with the subtitles but challenge yourself not to reply on the captioning exclusively. It's a good way to practice and will help with listening comprehension.
- YouTube has children's books with a reader. Storyonline.com is another excellent source for those beginning to rehab.
- Listen to audiobooks following along with the printed version of the book if helpful. Your local library may have an audiobook collection you can access for free.
- The Great Courses are lecture series on hundreds of topics. They may be found at your local library online. They are not closed captioned which forces you to lipread the lecturer while streaming the audio to your processor.
- Have someone read the newspaper or a passage from a book or poem and have you repeat it back to them.
- Have fun with your hearing rehab. Play games like name that sound. Enlist the help of family/friends to challenge you to name the sounds around you. Invent your own game.
- Listen to the radio (talk radio) when driving.
- If you don't have small children go to the park or playground to familiarize yourself with the way they speak.

- Have a child read to you or sing his/her favorite song. Children's voices can be just as difficult to understand as an adult's voice.
- Listen to music—easy listening/mellow—without a lot of instruments or vocals. Start by finding a song you remember following along with printed lyrics to jog your mental/listening memory. As you begin to understand music add different types of songs/music to your listening list. Hearmusicagain.com has helpful hints and easy listening internet music.
- Old songs may not sound like you remember them. In fact, they probably won't. Don't be discouraged. Your brain needs to learn to recognize them again. If the first time you listen to an old favorite, it sounds "off," play it again and again. Your brain will catch up to your ears! YouTube music videos of familiar sounds will help. Search for your favorite song and add the words: with lyrics to your search term. You brain will kick in faster with the lyrics and the music together. Remember, even people with normal hearing often have problems with understanding the lyrics. Patience will pay off.
- Music with more rhythm tends to be easier to learn. In the beginning, jazz with a lot of brass, is the easiest way to get music to sound recognizable and normal.
- Set up times to call family members and friends to hold a phone conversation every day.
- Go for a walk or sit outside to re-acclimate or learn the sounds of nature. Try to pick out the different songs that birds sing. Soon those songs will be in perfect harmony.

Additional Resources from Cochlear Implant Basics by Richard Pocker

- Go to restaurants at non-peak times.
- Turn on appliances such as the microwave, dishwasher, washer, dryer etc. Put your ear close to anything around the house just to learn the sound.
- Utilize your wireless accessories. They can be a big help in various situations (car, restaurant, etc.) Each manufacturer offers their own set of devices. Do your research. When doing rehabilitation exercises from a laptop or television, direct streaming of the sound source is preferred.
- Sit at the front of the room to hear/see the speaker. Don't be shy. If you cannot hear a speaker at a lecture or in a classroom, ask them to clip a remote mic accessory to their shirt or jacket. It will make the experience much more enjoyable. Just don't forget to get it back at the end.
- Use a T-Coil setting to help you hear in venues that are equipped with the hearing loop.
- Use your remote assistant. Adjust the volume and sensitivity for different hearing environments. Your audiologist can help you select settings that are suitable for your lifestyle and interests. Remember again, no two people have the same loss or the same solution for their hearing journey. Everyone can have a customized solution.
- **Think outside the box!!!** There is so much you can do to connect the dots to hearing. Just use your imagination.
- **Other helpful ideas:**
- Keep a journal of both good and bothersome issues you encounter. Take that journal to your appointments with your audiologist. This specific feedback will provide your

audiologist a better understanding of the problems you may be experiencing positively influence adjustments.

- Work with your audiologist to improve the fine tuning. Ask about T (threshold levels—softest sounds you hear) and C levels (comfort levels—loudest sounds you can comfortably tolerate). Discuss the different programs/coding strategies and when to use them. Learn as much as you can about the process and the features available to your processor.
- Manufacturers recommend that you change your microphone covers once every three months or sooner if you live in an area where humidity is high, you perspire often or notice a change in sound quality. Keeping clean microphone covers in place is important.
- Ideally, store your processor in a dryer such as a Zephyr or other drying device, every night. If your device has a replaceable desiccant cartridge be sure to mark the date on it and replace as per the instructions. REMEMBER: Moisture is the enemy of all electronics.
- If you use them, recharge your rechargeable batteries, and keep those not in use in the recharger unit.

Additional Resources from Cochlear Implant Basics by Richard Pocker

Useful Rehabilitation Programs and Support

- TED Talks www.ted.com/talks
- News in Easy English newsineasyenglish.com News in Easy English—Easy News for ESL Listening newsineasyenglish.com
- App called **Speech Banana**
- Practice phone calls with a family member or friend
- Audiobooks along with a print copy
- App called **Hear Coach**
- App called Nature Sounds
- App called **Breethe**
- App called **Coffitivity**
- App called **Mondly** for different languages
- App called **TOEIC** for English as a second language

Angel Sounds Interactive Listening Rehabilitation & Hearing test:
- http://angelsound.tigerspeech.com/

Aural Rehabilitation Resource Guide is another excellent source of programs, some free and others for sale. Aural-rehabiliation.pdf(unc.edu)

Facebook groups offer support for recipients of all ages. Some groups to consider are:
- Cochlear Implant Daily Rehab
- Bilateral CI Warrior
- Cochlear Awareness Network
- Cochlear Implant Users
- Cochlear Hybrid Implant Group
- Cochlear Implant Experiences
- Cochlear Implants How to Enjoy Music
- Podcast interviews at cochlearimplantbasics.com

These programs are produced by different cochlear implant manufacturers but may be utilized by other cochlear implant brand recipients.

COCHLEAR
- Communications Center
- http://www.cochlear.com/wps/wcm/connect/us/communication-corner

For a comprehensive Cochlear rehabilitation program, ask your Cochlear representative for the Adult-Home Based Hearing Therapy Manual (publication FUN3570 ISS2 Dept 20)

MED-EL
Rehab at home for adults' series

https://blog.medel.com/category/tips-tricks/rehab-at-home-posts/

Med-El Mondays aural rehabilitation small group zoom meetings.
They rotate topics each month, so all the topics show up and aural rehab is one of the topics.)

https://web.cvent.com/event/15c20e19-df0c-4dd7-b47f-2193f55b450b/regProcessStep1

Med-El adult rehabilitation kits to use with a family member or friend.

https://blog.medel.pro/introducing-medel-adult-rehabilitation-kits/

One on one captioned zoom meetings with a Med-El audiologist to help guide aural rehabilitation (aural rehab is one of the topics to select when registering for the free time slot)

Additional Resources from Cochlear Implant Basics by Richard Pocker

https://web.cvent.com/event/9f87401e-5bd8-4868-9e78-1fbba262e086/regProcessStep1

https://www.medel.com/support/rehab/rehabilitation-downloads

https://www.medel.com/support/rehab

Music For Cochlear Implant Users: MED-EL's Spotify Playlists - The MED-EL Blog (medel.com)

ADVANCED BIONICS
- https://hearingsuccess.com
- https://play.google.com/store/apps/details?id=com.advanced bionics.wordsuccess&hl=en_US&gl=US
- https://thelisteningroom.com
- https://www.advancedbionics.com/us/en/home/ab4kids/tool s-for-schools.html

Some Closing Comments about Rehabilitation
One of the most common areas of concern that candidates for a cochlear implant mention is rehabilitation. How much time is required for sounds to normalize? How many hours a day will they need to do it? What if they live alone and do not have a "hearing partner" to assist them. What programs are available?

All hearing journeys are unique. That also applies to rehabilitation. In rare cases, at activation, it all sounds normal. These "rockstar" activations are heartwarming, but most of us require effort to hear sounds as we remember.

Robin Chisholm Seymour's observation about rehabilitation says it best:
> "Although I do recognize and appreciate the existence of specialized apps and tools that are now available to recipients, I strongly believe that real life listening is necessary. My suggestion is that it

is so important to think about what you wanted to get cochlear implants and how being able to hear can impact your life in terms of work, interests, communications, etc. Not only are our CI learning journeys unique, but our motivations and goals are as well, as our interests and needs.

That being said, I've shared before that I got my first CI in early 2010, and there was no social media like today. We did not have wireless streaming with or without an accessory or hardware and we did not have any apps.

My personal goal was and continues to be that I live my life as normally and as fully as I used to prior to my hearing loss. I am not willing to compromise or give up anything in my life as a result of hearing challenges. My definition of those words, 'rehabilitation' or 'practice,' is much broader than in sometimes used. I believe that our brain has to learn to hear with the CI and has to learn to hear it within those environments that we are going to experience within the contents of our needs and interest.

What I did and continue to do is wear my Cis during all waking hours and in all hearing environments that I want to experience. The only streaming I do at all is to use the phone, which I do extremely easily and pretty much all day long. I don't use headphones. I don't use an accessory, and I do occasionally stream music. But I went from not being able to listen to music at all prior to my Cis, to pushing through music. Music sounded terrible. Gradually, overtime, it improved to the point that I now listen to music directly through whatever source is, radio, CD's and concerts, etc.

I had to hit the ground running after my first CI and that included working, volunteering, and most important horse shows which were extremely noisy as you can imagine. Going to dinner in a noisy restaurant at a huge table with 25 people obviously was challenging, but I still did it.

Additional Resources from Cochlear Implant Basics by Richard Pocker

> My learning to hear with my CI's. Has been challenging. Daily listening and exposing myself to the world sounds and speech, no matter initially how challenging it was. Because after my first CI I had no speech or sound or understanding at all. My audiologist gave me pages and pages of exercises to do, but those were list of individual words to practice with another person with a mouth covered so I could learn individual words. We graduated to simple sentences.
>
> I know that this can be done with an app, but I was listening to real voices rather than streaming. Having tools now. To help. With learning to hear with the CIs are wonderful. But it's also important to keep in mind it's going to take more than a couple of hours a day of rehab or practice with an app to get to feeling functional and comfortable out in the everyday world. My suggestions are to always identify your hearing goals, your life goals, and then adapt any learning strategy to those goals. They worked for me."

Kelly Flodin, another cochlear implant recipient, reiterated Robin's observations:

> "I agree with Robin that real life, real world listening, in all the environments we find ourselves in, is the best rehab for CIs. I consider anything we listen to as rehab. We want to hear what goes on around us in real life every day so actual practicing is critical, in my opinion.
>
> I've had my CIs for a little over two years. Early on I would just listen to the world around me and try tracking down and identifying anything I could hear. I got speech recognition pretty quickly. Conversations were the best for that."

Printed in the USA
CPSIA information can be obtained
at www.ICGtesting.com
CBHW052305301024
16686CB00009B/700